OVERCOMING TENDONITIS

A SYSTEMATIC APPROACH TO THE EVIDENCE-BASED TREATMENT OF TENDINOPATHY

STEVEN LOW, DPT
FRANK SKRETCH, DPT

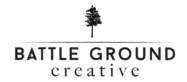

BATTLE GROUND
creative

Overcoming Tendonitis: A Systematic Approach to Evidence-Based Treatment of Tendinopathy

Published in Houston, Texas, by Battle Ground Creative
First Edition

ISBN: 978-1-947554-02-3 (softcover)
ISBN: 978-1-947554-03-0 (ebook)

HEALTH & FITNESS / Pain Management

Battle Ground Creative is a publishing company with an emphasis on helping first-time authors find their voice. Named after an obscure city in Washington State, we currently operate offices in Houston, Texas and Philadelphia, Pennsylvania. For a complete title list and bulk order information, please visit www.battlegroundcreative.com

The websites and references contained within this book are intended to serve as a resource with no guarantee expressed or implied as to the accuracy of their content.

Edited by Jared Stump
Cover design by Corinne Karl
Interior design and typeset by Katherine Lloyd

Printed in the United States of America

DISCLAIMER

By using *Overcoming Tendonitis* (hereafter referred to as "the book"), you (hereafter referred to as "the user"), signify your agreement to the following terms and conditions. If you do not agree to the terms and conditions outlined on this page, do not use this book!

- Material contained in the book is for educational purposes only. The authors, publisher, and other agents of the book assume no responsibility for any aspect of healthcare administered with the aid of content obtained from the book.

- In no case shall the authors, illustrators, editors, publisher, suppliers, or any other third party referenced be liable for any damages (both now and in the future) including, but not limited to: physical injuries to any part of the body or multiple parts of the body, non-physical damages such as emotional pain and financial loss, tendon pain or damage, muscle strains or tears, illness and disease, heart attack, death; however caused, occurring during or after the user's altering of their habits, actions, diet, exercise, and/or lifestyle based upon usage of the content provided by the book.

- The user's usage of any and all content provided within the book is at the user's own risk. This includes suggested workouts, exercises, rehabilitation routines, nutritional information, and all other information.

- User understands that any and all advice and suggested programs pertaining to tendons, rehabilitation, and exercise should be performed after consulting with the appropriate medical professionals, under the guidance of a qualified rehabilitation specialist.

- User understands nutritional advice is not intended as a substitute for professional medical advice, diagnosis, and/or treatment, and has been advised to seek medical advice from a physician before altering a diet or beginning an exercise program.

CONTENTS

INTRODUCTION

Tendonitis has been an interesting topic to research. When we looked at the efficacy of each treatment option for individual parts of the body, we were intrigued to find that the results varied. Treatments that worked slightly or moderately well for one form of tendonitis may work poorly or not at all for other types of tendonitis. Thus, as we reviewed the research, this book evolved from a big-picture look at different tendonitis treatment options to a specific integration of treatment options for different afflicted tendons.

As this book is a compilation of both research and expert opinions, we recommend that you talk to your doctor or medical professional before utilizing any of the information or suggestions presented in this book, as referenced in greater detail on the "disclaimer page." The primary reason for this is because the information in this book is presented in a generalized manner based on what tends to work best for most of the population as an aggregate. Generalized information can be effective in many circumstances; however, your medical professional may recognize subtleties and/or intricacies of your case that could drive them to avoid certain types of treatment, utilizing other methods instead. This tends to be more effective than generalized treatment. At the same time, if your medical practitioners are not aware of some of the more recent research relating to tendonitis, it could likely help with your treatment to share some of the things you learn through this book.

Additionally, this book will not contain information about the diagnosis of tendinopathy, as we have found that many patients and athletes are inclined to self-diagnose their own injuries rather than see the appropriate medical professional. When it comes to tendinopathy in particular, this self-diagnosis is often inaccurate due to the complexity of the issues involved. Even if the tendinopathy diagnosis is accurate, there could be other factors or issues with one's technique that is contributing to it.

We hope that incidents of self-diagnosis will decrease. Please understand that use of any of the information presented in this book, apart from proper diagnosis and instruction from a medical professional, is strictly "at your own risk" and, in many cases, ill-advised.

Most medical professionals understand that research and expert opinions are constantly evolving and changing over time. We have worked diligently to gather not only a great deal of information but *up-to-date* information. However, there may be evidence we have failed to cover. If a medical professional were to discover clinically effective information that is not covered in this book, it would be beneficial for both them and their clients to use their experience and critical thinking skills to integrate it into their treatment plans.

In short, this book is not intended to be the end-all of knowledge and treatment of tendonitis.

Personally, we like to integrate the strongest research evidence, barring any contraindications, into the treatment plans we provide to our patients. If it fails to help them, we modify the plan as needed, and also integrate treatment plans that have shown to only work slightly to moderately well for the general population, as they may be highly effective for a specific individual. Given that one often will utilize different lines of evidence and treatments simultaneously, it is important to be on the lookout for areas where you can add or subtract treatments as the patient progresses or declines. The patient is the priority, not "sticking to the plan."

Steven Low, DPT
Frank Skretch, DPT, CMTPT

CHAPTER 1

UNDERSTANDING THE LEVELS AND CLASSIFICATION OF EVIDENCE IN STUDIES

OVERVIEW OF LEVELS AND CLASSIFICATION OF EVIDENCE

Over the past ten to fifteen years, studies in physical therapy and other disciplines have begun classifying evidence according to various grades. This allows scientists to make more accurate observations about how scientific evidence may or may not apply to clinical guidelines and treatment. Below you will find a basic summary of how this evidence is classified for diagnostic, prospective, and therapeutic studies according to the Center for Evidence-Based Medicine.[1]

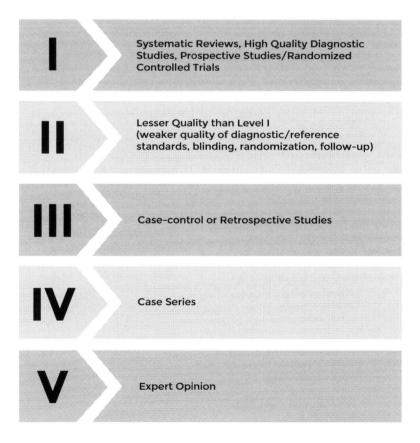

I — Systematic Reviews, High Quality Diagnostic Studies, Prospective Studies/Randomized Controlled Trials

II — Lesser Quality than Level I (weaker quality of diagnostic/reference standards, blinding, randomization, follow-up)

III — Case-control or Retrospective Studies

IV — Case Series

V — Expert Opinion

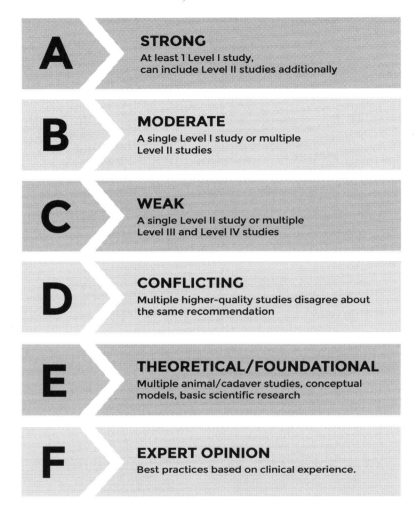

This evidence can be compiled into a grading system that moves from A-D. Furthermore, the inclusion of expert opinion and scientific theoretical evidence means there are six different levels from A-F. These indicate the relative strength of any recommendations for application to clinical viability.

Not all of these will be used everywhere within the first section. There is currently only one "gold standard" article utilizing the classifications of evidence for tendonitis. This is currently for Achilles tendonitis and it is called *Achilles Pain, Stiffness, and Muscle Power Deficits; Midportion Achilles Tendinopathy Revision.*[2]

OVERVIEW OF THE DECISION-MAKING PROCESS

The Achilles article referenced above includes a decision-making tree that can guide clinicians in all the phases of rehabilitation. These components are as follows:

1. Medical screening.
2. Classifying the condition.
3. Determining the irritability stage.
4. Selecting appropriate outcome measures.
5. Selecting appropriate interventional strategies.
6. Re-evaluating improvement and modification of strategies (if needed).

1: MEDICAL SCREENING

Physical therapy evaluation and intervention.

OR

Physical therapy along with consultation from another healthcare provider.

OR

Consultation with another healthcare provider only.

 REFER OUT

2: CLASSIFY CONDITION

Differential diagnosis through clinical findings.

Does patient examination suggest Achilles tendinopathy?

Consideration of other pain sources. (eg: lumbar radiculopathy, other systemic/medical conditions)

REFER OUT

3: IRRITABILITY STAGING

Decision if stage is acute or non-acute.

• Staging is important to guide clinical decisions of treatment frequency, duration, intensity, and type

• Use clinical judgment if irritability does not match symptom duration/presentation

4: OUTCOME MEASURES

Used to assess level of functioning, associated impairments, response to treatment.

Most commonly used for Achilles tendinopathy:
   • VISA-A, FAAM, LEFS
   • VAS Pain Scale
   • Range of motion, maual muscle testing, gait testing

5: INTERVENTION STRATEGIES

Determine acute vs. non-acute diagnostic indicators to guide intervention strategies.

Common intervention examples:
   • Modalities, taping, other passive treatment
   • Stretching, eccentric loading exercises, neuromuscular education
   • Joint and soft-tissue mobilization

6: RE-EVALUATE

GOALS MET

NOT IMPROVING

DISCHARGE TO SELF-MANAGEMENT

REFERRAL TO OTHER HEALTH PROVIDERS

Summary of Recommendations for Midportion Achilles Tendinopathy

DIAGNOSIS/CLASSIFICATION

C
- arc sign
- Royal London Hospital test
- gradual onset of pain subjectively reported 2-6cm proximal to Achilles tendon insertion
- pain with palpation of mid-portion of the Achilles tendon

EXAMINATION

A Outcome Measures: Activity Limitations/
Self-Reported Measure
- VISA-A for pain and stiffness
- FAAM or LEFS for functional limitations

B Activity Limitations/
Physical Performance Measures
- hop test
- heel-raise endurance test

B Physical Impairment Measures
- ankle dorsiflexion and subtalar ranges of motion
- plantar flexion strength and endurance
- static arch height and forefoot alignment
- pain with palpation

INTERVENTIONS

GOLD STANDARD INTERVENTION

A Exercise in the form of mechanical loading of tendon using eccentric or concentric/eccentric guided programs

INTERVENTIONS TO CONSIDER

B Patient education and activity modification without complete cessation (within pain tolerance)

B Iontophoresis for pain reduction in acute cases only

C Stretching

F Patient counseling about key factors involved with condition

F Neuromuscular Re-education

F Manual Therapy

F Dry needling in combination with eccentric exercises with symptoms lasting over three months

F Rigid taping for reducing tendon strain and alter foot mechanics

INTERVENTIONS WITH CONTRADICTORY EVIDENCE: NO RECOMMENDATION CAN BE MADE

D Heel Lifts

D Orthoses

E Low-level Laser Therapy

INTERVENTIONS THAT ARE NOT RECOMMENDED

C Night Splints

F Elastic taping attempting to reduce pain or improve function

CHAPTER 2

UNDERSTANDING THE TENDINOPATHY PROCESS

A BRIEF HISTORY OF TENDINOPATHY

Tendonitis was the traditional term used to describe the disorder of the tendon due to perceived inflammatory reaction in acute cases of dysfunction (the *-itis* suffix is the medical term for inflammation). In 1976, Puddu first used the term *tendinosis* to describe the abnormal state of degeneration of the tendon in athletes that was persistent[3]. This was when histological (microscopic) evidence showed there was little to no inflammation associated with the progressive tendon disorder compared to the traditional term tendonitis.[4,5] Finally, in the late 1990s, Maffuli et al desired to shift clinical terminology from tendonitis/tendinosis to tendinopathy in order to avoid confusion with both terms.[6] Unfortunately, much of the confusion still exists today, even in the medical community.

Tendinopathy has since become the preferred term by those in the scientific research field to refer to the spectrum of dysfunction and pain associated with the tendon, paratendon, and surrounding structures—including the various stages such as reactive and degenerative tendinopathy.[7, 8] However, the term *tendonitis* is still commonly used by most people, even some healthcare practitioners. Other common terms such as *medial epicondylitis* (colloquially *golfer's elbow*) or *lateral epicondylitis* (colloquially *tennis elbow*) are misnomers as the *-itis* ending denotes an inflammatory response which is absent or minimally present and conflicts with the traditional healing model. Because of this, the verbiage has shifted to medial or lateral tendinopathy. Alternatively, some have begun to describe the tendinopathy by the area of pain, such as medial or lateral epicondylalgia (as *the -algia* suffix denotes pain) since tendinopathy usually presents with spot pain directly on and/or in the tendon.[9]

We will primarily use the term *tendinopathy* throughout this book, as the terms *tendonitis* and *epicondylitis* are incorrect for our purposes. We decided to use the former in the title of the book because this is still the common term most people associate with tendinopathy.

Medical professionals have a difficult time understanding the various stages of tendinopathy and their different presentations. There are several different tendinopathy models that have appeared in scientific literature over time, each of which have their different merits. We will examine them sequentially to get a good picture of what is occurring in the tendinopathy process.

TENDINOPATHY MODELS

A 2007 model by Arnoczky et al proposed that tendon problems may be the result of overstimulation, though sometimes occasionally understimulation, of the tendon.[10]

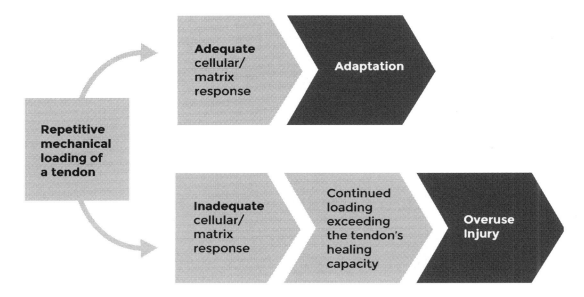

Overstimulation of the tendon is the most obvious as tendinopathy is generally considered an overuse injury, but understimulation can occur via atrophy from too much rest or in late-stage degeneration. This model was limited in explaining much of the cause and effect, symptoms, or process of rehabilitation of tendinopathy, but it got the ball rolling.

The Iceberg model, proposed in 2009 by Abate et al, began to examine the process of tendinopathy and attempted to categorize it into various stages.[11]

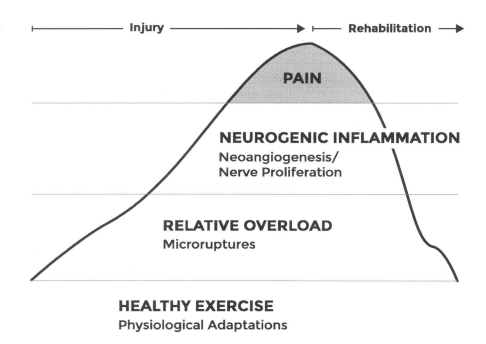

The Iceberg model attempted to show the process of overload dysfunction, even before pain begins to appear in the tendon. Overloaded, dysfunctional tendons were thought to have micro ruptures that potentially led to disruption of the tendon, resulting in the nerves being affected, which caused pain. This was a very limited model of explaining the entire process.

In the same year, Cook and Purdam proposed that tendinopathy dysfunction progression should be thought of as a continuum, also taking place in various stages.[12]

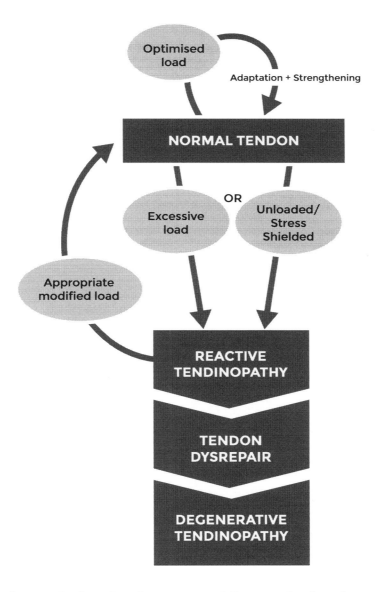

The Cook and Purdam study describes the conceptual framework of tendinopathy development. This was an important study because it showed that tendons tend to react differently to various methods of rehabilitation depending on the stage of tendinopathy.

The failed healing model, proposed in 2010 by Fu et al, began to integrate many of the histological (microscopic) changes that were seen in overuse tendinopathy.[13]

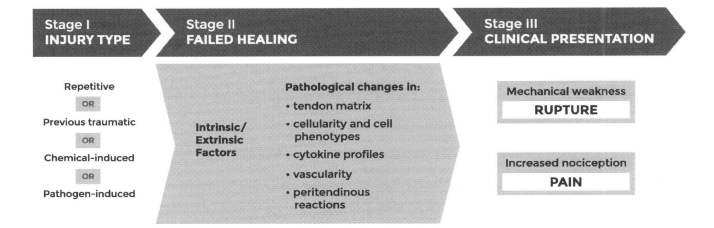

Finally, as their research progressed, Cook et al published another update to their model in 2016. This revised model covers more of the variables associated with dysfunctional tendons.[14] It explains how pain, pathology, and function interact as the tendon progresses through the continuum.

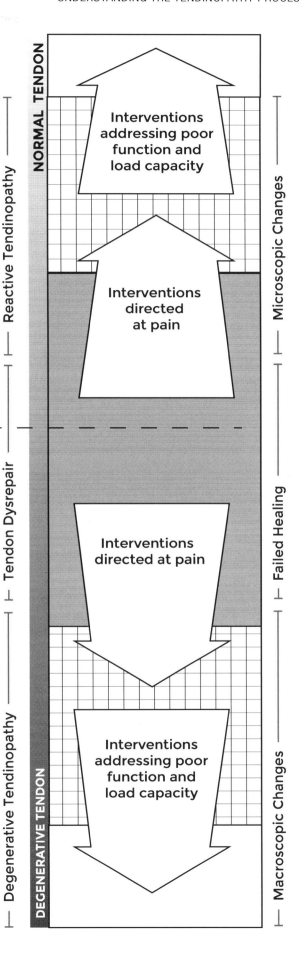

STATE OF PAIN & FUNCTION

- The pain-free tendon with good function
- The pain-free tendon with poor function/ insufficient load capacity
- The painful tendon with poor function

Likelihood of structure returning to normal

- - - - - - - - - - - - -

Limited ability to remodel tendon structure

Reactive-on-degenerative tendinopathy occurs when some part of the tendon is already degenerative.

The tendon is still being overloaded which can cause some of the normal tendon surrounding the degenerative portion to become reactive.

Reactive Tendinopathy

Tendon Dysrepair

Degenerative Tendinopathy

NORMAL TENDON

DEGENERATIVE TENDON

Interventions addressing poor function and load capacity

Interventions directed at pain

Interventions directed at pain

Interventions addressing poor function and load capacity

Microscopic Changes

Failed Healing

Macroscopic Changes

To put this in context, a normal tendon is comprised of approximately 90 percent type I collagen, in a cross-linked triple helix structure, with water molecules stabilizing with hydrogen bonds.[15, 16] For the layman, this is like the DNA double helix except with three strands of collagen wrapping around each other instead of two strands of DNA. These structures are then replicated parallel to one other to form bigger structures of fibrils, fibers, and fascicles that are connected to proteoglycans.[17] This is similar to muscle fiber structure, which is made up of smaller bundles organized into larger bundles.

We can integrate the Cook et al and Fu et al models to get an idea of the various pathological changes in the tendon as it progresses through these stages. You will find the layman's explanation in parentheses below:

- If limited inflammation → Pro-inflammatory cytokines (possible pain and healing response).
- Neovascularization → Hypervascularity (increase in blood vessel growth).
- Innervation → Increased neuropeptides and innervation (nerve in-growth into the tendon).
- Cell recruitment/apoptosis → hypercellularity, increased apoptosis (cell death).
- Matrix synthesis → Mucoid, lipoid, calcific degeneration (abnormal changes, such as fatty or calcified tendon).
- Tenogenic differentiation/apoptosis → Mucoid, lipoid, calcific degeneration (abnormal changes, such as fatty or calcified tendon).
- Matrix remodeling → Collagenolysis, tendon adhesion (collagen breakdown and the tendon functions worse).

Here are some additional common changes that contribute to the weakened structure and function of a degenerative tendon:

- Vasculature around the tendon becomes malformed or irregular.[18]
- Type I collagen is replaced by weaker type III collagen, and the collagen arrangement becomes disordered and weaker.[19-20]
- Increases in ground substance may lead to a lack of collagen or collagen breakdown.[21]
- Neurotransmitters, such as glutamate, which may be potentially responsible for pain signaling are present in tendons with chronic pain.[22]
- Aside from mucoid, lipoid, and calcific changes in some tendons there can also be hypoxic, hyaline, myxoid, fibrinoid with fibrocartilaginous or osseous metaplasia changes.[23-24]
- For some visuals, Riley histologically examines healthy tendons and contrasts them to pathological tendons in *Tendon and ligament biochemistry and pathology.*[25]

An important thing of note is that the variety of pathological changes in the tendon vary widely, especially when moving from the reactive stage to the dysrepair and degenerative stages. This may be one of the reasons why there is a lot of variability in outcomes in tendinopathy rehabilitation. For example, some tendons exhibit the *osseus metaplasia*, which is synonymous with the term of *calcification*, resulting in calcific tendinopathy. One type of tendon with certain degenerative changes may not respond as well as tendons with other degenerative changes.

TENDINOPATHY STAGING

Joseph et al goes on to summarize the process in which all of these changes take place within the Cook continuum model.[26] This clarifies when many of the pathological changes are occurring in each of the continuum stages.

Reactive tendinopathy is proposed to occur in response to acute overload and is described as a noninflammatory, proliferative response. In vitro work supports this observation of hypercellularity, absence of inflammatory infiltrate, and the shift toward synthesis of large modular prostaglandins.

Tendon dysrepair or *failed healing* is the second stage of the continuum proposed by Cook and Purdam, which resembles the initial stage of reactivity but with greater matrix disorganization. Neovascularity and neuronal ingrowth occur and represent an aspect of attempted, but failed, repair. Evidence exists that the tendon can recover in both form and function from this stage with appropriate treatment that includes load modulation and eccentric exercise stimulus.

Degenerative tendinopathy (tendinosis) is the final stage in this continuum. Features include vast areas of hypocellularity, pooling of proteoglycan, and severely disorganized collagen. It is thought that these changes are largely irreversible.

From a clinical perspective, this model divides tendinopathy into two distinct groups: early reactive and late dysrepair/degeneration. Local swelling and mildly focal hypoechoic lesions on ultrasound in a younger individual indicate early reactive tendinopathy. A thick nodular tendon with large defined areas of hypoechogenicity and evidence of vascular ingrowth typically identified in older individuals represents late degenerative tendinopathy. In either clinical picture, symptoms can be variable and occur at any point in the continuum.

Understanding this process is important because it shows us that some tendon changes that are seemingly contradictory are actually not, such as hypercellularity (increase in tendon cells) and hypocellularity (decrease in tendon cells). They are simply progressions in the continuum model. In the reactive stage, where the tendon is attempting to adapt to the load, it makes sense that there is an increase of cells trying to adapt to the load. However, with continued overload, this may result in negative changes like cell apoptosis (cell death), which happen as the tendon progresses poorly from the reactive stage to dysrepair and, finally, the degenerative stage.

This is the clearest overall picture of tendinopathy we have currently, which should help both medical professionals and patients understand that pain, pathology, and function are not necessarily one in the same. In most cases, there is an increase in pain, pathology, and loss of function as the stages progress. However, that is not always the case. Sometimes, there is only poor function. Other times, there is a degenerative, non-painful tendon with poor function, or there could be a degenerative, non-painful tendon with good function. Up to 85-90 percent of Achilles tendon ruptures may happen without signs of pain, swelling, and stiffness,[27,28] though there are usually other predisposing factors that may increase risk of injury. One example would be intense intermittent activity, such as with weekend warriors.

Overall, any interventions that are used in tendinopathy should be addressed to the stage the tendon is in, both for pain and function. We will discuss this extensively in subsequent chapters.

INTRINSIC AND EXTRINSIC RISK FACTORS

Morgan and Coetzee did a study on the various intrinsic and extrinsic factors in developing patellar tendinopathy, as illustrated in the image below.[29]

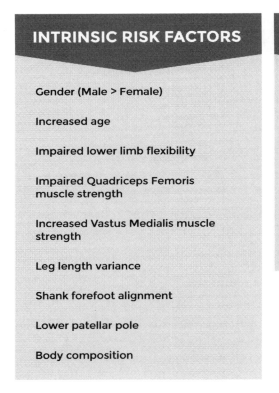

INTRINSIC RISK FACTORS	EXTRINSIC RISK FACTORS
Gender (Male > Female)	Hard physical work in combination with jumping sports
Increased age	Heavy physical demanding work in volleyball and basketball players
Impaired lower limb flexibility	Physical activity
Impaired Quadriceps Femoris muscle strength	Type of sport: Jumping sport
Increased Vastus Medialis muscle strength	Level of sports participation (elite vs recreational)
Leg length variance	
Shank forefoot alignment	
Lower patellar pole	
Body composition	

In every case of tendinopathy, both intrinsic and extrinsic factors are typically present. They can be used to:

- Help screen those who have a greater propensity to develop tendinopathy as an overuse injury.
- Assist in screening athletes and patients who currently have tendinopathy in order to understand that they may need to modify certain external factors and progress more slowly in rehabilitation and after rehabilitation if they have more risk factors than others.

While we will not cover all of the intrinsic and extrinsic risk factors for the different variations of tendinopathy, there are many common risk factors in every variation, which include: sex, age, obesity, variance in strength (weakness, in particular), impaired flexibility (less than normal range of motion), and body structure are very common intrinsic risk factors for most lower-body tendinopathy. Likewise, many extrinsic risk factors can be profession-related (repetitive strain due to repetitive tasks) and often overuse-related such as level of sport, impacts in sport, and combinations of excessive volume, frequency, or intensity in exercise.

These generalized indicators are something that you can look for in all forms of tendinopathy. Other common indicators are technique-related or compensation-related due to pain or otherwise poor technique. This is where a medical professional (like a physical therapist) can help you evaluate your lifestyle or exercise to examine different areas that could possibly be contributing toward developing or exacerbating tendinopathy.

TENDINOPATHY, REHABILITATION, AND OUTCOMES

According to the Cook et al study, only a portion of a tendon with tendinopathy is reactive/dysrepair, reactive on degenerative, or degenerative. This has been confirmed through both ultrasound and magnetic resonance imaging (MRI) studies.[30-31] As rehabilitation progresses, tendinopathy in the dysrepair stage and degenerative portions of the tendon will likely become more asymptomatic and be able to function to some degree, while the healthy tendon can compensate for the rest.

COMMON FLEXOR TENDON AS A WHOLE

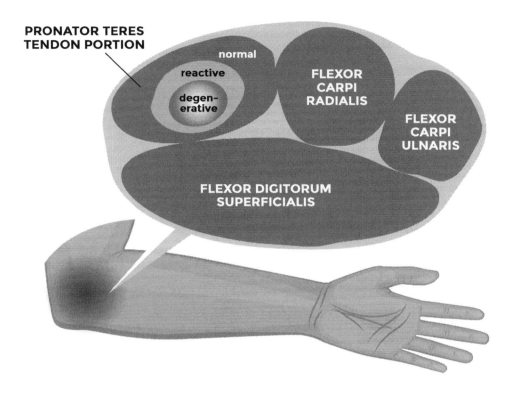

Reactive-on-degenerative tendinopathy can be common in those who have had tendinopathy for several months or years. Typically, there will be some portion of the tendon that is degenerative but other portions will be reactive. Rest may help clear up the reactive portion, but any progress made will eventually stall because the degenerative portion will not improve with either function or pain with rest. Therefore, focused rehabilitation is important to improve the function of the healthy parts of the tendon. As load tolerance increases, the degenerative portion will typically become more asymptomatic and less painful.

Scientific literature on MRI studies in other populations reveals that degeneration is common throughout the population, even as many of those in the degenerative stage have no symptoms of their degeneration, such as pain. A systematic review by Brinjikji et al found that disc degeneration "increased from 37 percent of 20-year-old individuals to 96 percent of 80-year-old individuals" and similar percentages were found with disc bulges, disc protrusions, and annular fissures without the presence of pain.[32]

Similarly, degeneration in tendons is common. Kannus et al looked at the incidence of degeneration of tendons during autopsy and found that 34 percent showed signs of degeneration.[33] The prevalence of Achilles tendinopathy may be about 6 percent in the sedentary population and as high as 50 percent in elite athletes.[34] Asymptomatic Achilles tendinopathy under ultrasound examination may range from about 4 to 16 percent or more based on some studies.[35,36] In the case of diabetes, the incidence of asymptomatic Achilles tendinopathy was about 25 percent vs. 12 percent in the normal population.[37] Even signs of various stages of tendinopathy on imaging may not correlate with presentation of the tendinopathy in rehabilitation or symptoms like pain.[38]

Indeed, a 2019 review by Docking and Cook acknowledges that there is a high rate of asymptomatic pathological tendons along with increasing evidence that structural changes, such as tendon remodeling or repair, are not necessary for positive clinical outcomes.[39]

This is important for both medical professionals and patients to understand. Much of the time, tendinopathy in some of the more severe stages like degenerative or reactive on degenerative can still be treated through rehabilitation and progress to the point where one can perform daily activities and even resume sports with little or no pain. Many patients who have had tendinopathy for several months or even years will start feeling down or hopeless; thus, it can be helpful for their psychological wellbeing to educate them regarding proper rehabilitation. In fact, this could provide them with motivation to pursue such rehabilitation.

While the stage of tendinopathy may help a medical professional outline a patient's plan for rehabilitation, it should not be misused by either party to essentially determine a prognosis that is inconsistent with the evidence.

Blazina was one of the first to propose clinical grading systems for evaluating tendinopathy.[40] However, practice has evolved over time to use various outcome measures that can accurately track improvement in pain and function rather than specific staging. Different clinical outcome measures are used for different tendinopathies. For instance, the gold standard article for Achilles tendinopathy[41] recommends that the VISA-A[42] be used in conjunction with either the FAAM[43] or LEFS[44] to see if different interventions are working during treatment. We will discuss these in the final chapter of this book.

CHAPTER 3

COMMON MYTHS
OF TENDINOPATHY

Now that we have examined the science surrounding the development and stages of tendinopathy, let's take a look at a few of the common myths we often hear pertaining to tendinopathy recovery and rehabilitation.

REST

One common treatment you may encounter for diagnosed tendinopathy will simply be to "rest." This advice may come from doctors, physical therapists, coaches, friends, or family members. However, it is not consistent with current research.

As we can see from the tendinopathy models in the previous chapter, rest is only effective when there is reactive tendinopathy or reactive on degenerative tendinopathy (for the reactive portion). Cessation of the workouts or exercises that have been aggravating the tendinopathy allows the tendon to heal some on its own. In the case of reactive on degenerative, it will improve to a certain point and then stop due to the reactive portion clearing up while the degenerative portion remains.

Rest typically does not work for tendinopathy within progressive dysrepair or degenerative stages, as the tendons in those stages have deleterious changes that are thought to be largely irreversible. However, these irreversible changes are only limited to the small portions that are degenerative. Rehabilitation exercise helps build up load tolerance and improves function of the healthy portions of tendon. If resting does not help your diagnosed tendinopathy, then it's likely that there are some degenerative aspects that require rehabilitation exercise.

Please note that rest helps *diagnosed* forms of tendinopathy that are in the reactive or early dysrepair stages, but not degenerative tendinopathy. Self-diagnosis can be inaccurate in many cases, as similar problems can occur within an area that appear to be tendinopathy when they actually are not.

Diagnosis of tendinopathy is usually based on localized symptoms and presentation of function (or dysfunction), along with screening and differential diagnosis protocols by medical professionals. Symptoms may not necessarily correlate to the possible stage the tendon is in, which makes things trickier. Typically, only large-scale, degenerative changes can be seen on an ultrasound or MRI, which can be inconvenient, time-consuming, and expensive to obtain. Regardless, pinpointing a specific stage is generally not needed, as conservative treatment (e.g. physical therapy) is the recommended initial response to all forms of tendinopathy, despite the stage. However, a general understanding of stages can be used to make sure the exercise loading of the tendon is managed well. It is also important to evaluate if some of the possible symptoms (such as pain) are more acute or chronic, which can affect the approach of the tendinopathy needs to be treated. This will be discussed in Chapter 5.

ICE

Ice, especially in the *RICE* protocol (Rest, Ice, Compression, Elevation) is not particularly useful. Ice is typically used for acute injuries to decrease inflammation, reduce pain, and decrease blood flow or swelling.

If a tendon is in the reactive tendinopathy stage, then simple rest or removal of the aggravating exercises will help resolve the issue; no ice is needed. If the tendon is in the dysrepair or degenerative stage, there will still be little to no inflammation present (as tendinopathy is a non-inflammatory proliferation disorder) in the injured portion of the tendon. Since ice is used to decrease inflammation, there is no need for it. Rehabilitation exercises are much more useful for tendinopathy.

Additionally, ice has also been shown to decrease strength and muscle adaptations in cold water immersion studies.[45,46] While this does not show that there is potential for decreases in collagen synthesis rates in tendons, there is a possible mechanism here.

Many athletes swear by ice baths. These may potentially help them due to the large volumes of effort their body may need to decrease systemic inflammation to a more manageable level. The ice bath may simply make them feel better, even if there are actually negative physiological changes. However, this is not the case with tendinopathy since there is little to no inflammation in every stage.

As for the reduction in pain, analgesics are superior to ice as ice tends to decrease only surface-level pain. We will discuss analgesics a bit more in the next section. As for blood flow, we will also discuss that myth in the bullet point afterward.

If ice does help resolve the "tendinopathy," then it might not be tendinopathy in the first place. It could be another diagnosis like paratendonitis (inflammation of the tendon sheath), which can often seem like it is tendinopathy as it affects similar areas and tissues. It is common for some areas like the sub-acromial space around the rotator cuff, infrapatellar fat pad area, Achilles insertion area, and other areas of high compression to seem like tendinopathy but also be affecting other tissues where decreasing inflammation could be useful. It could be the case that one could have both tendinopathy and have the surrounding locations affected as well. Thus, decreases in inflammation or swelling may help, but they will help the surrounding areas and not the tendon itself. One common example is De Quervain's tenosynovitis where there can be tendinopathy but also swelling and inflammation of the tendon sheath.

In most cases, the RICE protocol is less effective than the newer *MEAT* protocol (Movement, Exercise, Analgesia, and Treatment). The RICE approach is the traditional model for injury treatment. The MEAT approach is an alternative model that is basically physical therapy rehabilitation in disguise. It is important to note that, in the MEAT approach, physical therapy is indicated from day one or even day zero. If you have had a knee replaced or sprained your ankle, the earlier you can begin physical therapy the better, as it will promote faster healing.

We rarely use or recommend the RICE approach anymore, even for acute injuries like a sprained ankle (assuming there are no catastrophic issues like torn ligaments or broken bones). Rest is obviously not good for a sprained ankle. You want as much early movement (within your pain tolerance level) as you can get. Slow movement within your range of motion will decrease your pain in many cases. Immobilizing the area leads to significantly longer recovery times because your muscles begin to stiffen up and the quality of your motor control decreases.

The use of ice is hotly debated. In practice, if there is no significant swelling taking place, ice is unnecessary. If there is swelling, compression is more effective than ice. Ice is really only useful for dulling pain, and analgesics usually do this more effectively. If you use compression, elevation is also unnecessary. Based on these factors, the RICE approach seems to be outdated and inferior to the MEAT approach.

ANALGESICS

There is some debate about whether or not to use NSAID (non-steroidal anti-inflammatory drug) pain relievers like ibuprofen for tendinopathy in any stage.

Like the trend we saw with cold water immersion, analgesics like ibuprofen (ex: Advil, Motrin) and paracetamol (ex: Tylenol, acetaminophen) have also shown negative impacts on the development of muscle protein synthesis (muscle hypertrophy) and strength gains.[47,48] As with ice, the potential for decrease in collagen synthesis rates is also present with some analgesics.

One possible use of analgesics for tendinopathy may be when the tendon is in a reactive state and has been aggravated. Although there may not be as much inflammation in the tendon itself, the potential reduction of pain, and possibly swelling, of the areas around the tendon may help. Like ice, it must be noted that if analgesics do help resolve the tendinopathy, it might not be tendinopathy you are dealing with in the first place. It may instead be something like paratendonitis (inflammation of the tendon sheath, which can often seem like it is tendinopathy as both affect similar areas and tissues.

Isometric exercises have proven to be effective for managing tendinopathy pain, without the potential downsides of ice or analgesics. We will discuss them in Chapter 5.

PAIN

You may have heard that you shouldn't push through *painful exercises* because pain is bad. This is false. The reality is that you shouldn't push through *aggravating exercises*.

The difference between painful and aggravating exercises is simple. While some exercises may be painful in the moment, they yield a positive, progressive result over the course of a few sessions. These exercises, while painful, are beneficial to the rehabilitation process due to increasing load tolerance and function over time which often leads to a reduction in pain as well. On the other hand, sometimes non-painful exercises may lead toward further degeneration. One typical example is when an athlete is starting to develop tendon pain that continues to get worse over time but can warm up with exercise to the point that it "feels fine." So, they continue training rigorously thinking it will go away. In many of these cases, it will continue to get worse leading to less load tolerance and greater tendon dysfunction. It is best to remove these "aggravating exercises" (or similarly decrease intensity or volume) that lead to decreased performance, increased pain, and greater signs and symptoms of progressive tendinopathy.

Thus, it is not so much *pain* that we should be concerned about, but improving load tolerance and function over time. Exercises and training intensity or volume that decrease performance and increase signs and symptoms of tendinopathy (usually along with increasing pain) need to be removed or adjusted. Yet, painful exercises can be an applicable, and often necessary, part of the rehabilitation process when managed well.

Pain is generally correlative in an acute injury to an aggravating exercise but may not necessarily be associated with a chronic injury that lasts three to six months or more. Therefore, rehabilitative exercises should usually be performed under the supervision or treatment plan of a qualified medical professional. It can be risky to perform self-rehabilitation. Do so at your own risk.

This topic will be discussed more extensively in Chapter 5.

BLOOD FLOW

Another common misnomer of tendinopathy is that increasing blood flow aids in the rehabilitation process. We also believed this previously, but research has shown the opposite is true when it comes to tendinopathy.

Tendons affected by tendinopathy swell slightly, which can be verified by an ultrasound or MRI.[49] This is due to some of the abnormalities like neovascularization (e.g. ingrowth of blood vessels and nerves into the tendon), which we discussed in the previous chapter. This occurs due to cytokine and growth factor secretion.[50]

Angiogenesis occurs as part of the spectrum of pathology in tendinosis. This formation of new blood vessels is mediated by the cytokines: vascular endothelial growth factor (VEGF), interleukin-Ib (IL Ib), and tumor necrosis factor a (TNFa). Cytokines are secreted proteins of small, molecular weight that act locally and mediate communication between cells. VEGF expression is induced by hypoxia, and the region around rotator cuff tears is known to be ischemic. These cytokines are known to be involved with tissue inflammation, but in tendinosis they do not appear to be secreted by the cells classically associated with inflammation (neutrophils, macrophages, and lymphocytes). They may instead be secreted by fibroblasts located in the subacromial bursa.

The swelling and neovascularization are not necessarily related to pain or clinical symptoms.[51] Although the neurovascular ingrowth may not be the actual cause of pain and symptoms, eccentrics and resistance training seem to destroy them, which helps to normalize blood flow.[52] Thus, modalities such as heat, ice, or contrast baths will not affect this process. Voodoo flossing also falls under this category because of proposed increased blood flow. It may be helpful or neutral as far as joint mobilization and potentially breaking chronic pain patterns.

We personally like utilizing heat with the tendon, but not because it increases blood flow or aids in healing. Instead, it helps to decrease tendon stiffness and warms it up for rehabilitation exercises. It also has a similar pain-reducing effect similar to ice, without all the negative side effects.[53]

CHAPTER 4

TENDINOPATHY AND GENERAL REHABILITATION KNOWLEDGE

COLLAGEN SYNTHESIS AND TENDON LOADING FREQUENCY, INTENSITY, AND VOLUME

Magnusson et al provides a schematic showing, below approximately thirty hours, the net collagen synthesis is negative directly after exercise because collagen degradation outpaces synthesis.[54]

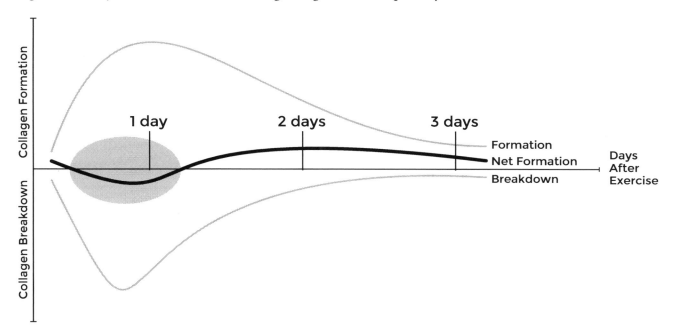

Therefore, it may not be a good idea to do continuous days of rehabilitation on an irritated tendon that is reactive or degenerative. This should be taken with a grain of salt because the variety of rehabilitation loading programs have different stimuli that accompany the frequency, such as a variety in intensity of the exercises or the total volume of the exercises.

Magnusson et al provides another chart that shows the response of collagen to loading at different intensity and volumes of exercise.

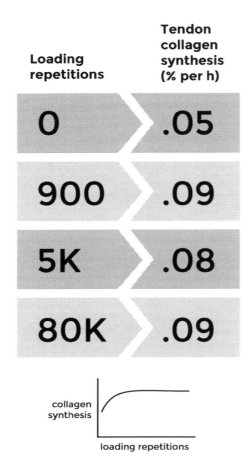

This chart shows a ceiling on the collagen synthesis. It shows that the loading response of 10 sets of 10 repetitions of knee extensions at 70 percent 1 Repetition Maximum (RM) is very similar to the loading response of 36 km of running. A lower-intensity activity such asmaximal knee kicking without resistance for 1 hour provides a similar collagen response as both of the above exercises.

Logically, a loading program that utilizes sufficient intensity and volume should be able to maximize collagen synthesis without an extreme amount of time commitment, such as 1 hour of knee kicking or 36 km of running, which could aggravate a reactive or degenerative tendon more than a standard loading program.

We see a similar concept with frequency of exercise in some studies. Alfredson,[55] Stanish and Curwin,[56] and Silbernagel[57] are some of the common Achilles loading programs that feature daily or even twice-a-day exercise. In these programs, the volume of the exercise is low enough that the frequency is well-tolerated, even if some of the programs are less effective than others.

Some evidence suggests that structural changes within the tendon shown on imaging do not explain the therapeutic improvements of exercise, except possibly in the case of heavy slow resistance.[58] It seems that the benefit of the therapeutic exercise actually comes from the removal of the aggravating exercise(s) (e.g. the particular exercise at too high intensity, volume, or frequency) and adaptation of the tendon, despite what stage it is in, to proper loading. The healthy portions of the tendon can have a positive training effect, and any degenerative portions can become asymptomatic. This agrees with the Docking and Cook review mentioned in previous chapters. Therefore, catering a rehabilitation program toward optimizing collagen synthesis may not be necessary to regain performance and decrease pain in a pathological tendon, but it will not be detrimental, either. It is worth considering as a small part of a program.

ECCENTRICS VS. CONCENTRIC-ECCENTRIC TRAINING

First off, allow us to provide a brief explanation regarding these terms. *Eccentric* is the name for the muscle-lengthening portion of an exercise (such as slowly lowering in a pushup or pull-up). The triceps and biceps muscles are lengthening in these respective movements. The *concentric* portion is the muscle-shortening or muscle contraction portion of the movement. This is when you push up from the bottom of a pushup, and when you pull your chin up to the bar from the bottom of the pull-up. Some of the first studies on Achilles tendinopathy used *only* eccentric training (slowly lowering from the top of a calf raise) as opposed to doing the full calf raise up and down consecutively.

Because eccentric training seems to be the most effective, we have heard it said that rehabilitation programs should only contain eccentrics. However, we find this to be short-sighted. If your goal is to return to your sport or resume daily activities, the concentric movement (whether controlled or explosive) is critical. Couppe et al analyzed this and concluded that isolated eccentric loading is likely no better than combined loading, though there is a limited amount of evidence to support this theory.[59]

> There is no convincing clinical evidence to demonstrate that isolated eccentric loading exercise improves clinical outcomes more than other loading therapies. However, the great variation and sometimes insufficient reporting of the details of treatment protocols may hamper the interpretation of what may be the optimal exercise regime with respect to parameters such as load magnitude, speed of movement, and recovery period between exercise sessions.

Some newer, randomized, controlled trials in lateral elbow tendinopathy by Stasinopoulus et al suggest that a combination of *all* the different contractions is the most effective method, though more studies are needed.[60]

> The eccentric-concentric training combined with isometric contractions was the most effective treatment. Future well-designed studies are needed to confirm the results of the present trial.

This would seem to make the most sense, given that isometrics effectively deal with pain and that combined eccentric and concentric training is necessary to prepare a patient to return to their sport, an occupation, or daily activities.

There is also some evidence from Bohm et al that tendon adaptation may primarily depend on loading intensity rather than type of muscle contraction.[61] This may mean performing an "eccentric" may not matter as much as a tendon getting enough load for adaptation. A longer eccentric contraction may have been enough intensity and volume for adaptation compared to the loading programs that were previously used. A potential corroborating fact from this study is that plyometric loading received mixed responses, which would make sense as the "short loading duration during jumping constrains the transduction of the mechanical stimulus" or, in other words, the limited loading period results in a lack of adaptation of the tendon. This seems to be the case, at least for isometric contractions.[62]

Overall, we think that going with a controlled eccentric *with* concentric repetition is likely the most effective way to maximize control and volume during rehabilitation. As you get further along in the rehabilitation stages, you can speed up the eccentric and concentric contractions in order to facilitate strength, power, and plyometric abilities, especially when returning an athlete to a sport.

PROGRAMMING, MODIFICATIONS TO ACTIVITY, AND ANALYSIS OF CURRENT RESEARCH

A 2013 Malliares et al systematic review looked at the different rehabilitation loading programs.[63] As mentioned previously, four of the most commonly used loading programs featured in scientific literature are the Alfredson, Stanish and Curwin, Silbernagel combined loading, and heavy-slow resistance (HSR).

PROGRAMS	TYPE OF EXERCISE	SETS, REPS	FREQUENCY	PROGRESSION	PAIN
Alfredson	Eccentric	3, 15	Twice daily	Load	Enough load to achieve up to moderate pain
Stanish and Curwin	Eccentric-concentric, power	3, 10-15	Daily	Speed then load	Enough load to be painful in the 3rd set
Silbernagel	Eccentric-concentric, eccentric, faster eccentric	Various	Daily	Volume, type of exercise	Acceptable if within defined limits
HSR	Eccentric-concentric	4, 15-6	3x/week	15-6 RM	Acceptable if was not worse after

The 2013 Malliares chart shows the variety of exercise rehabilitation loading programs.

To get an idea of the differences in loading sets and repetitions at a certain frequency, progression, and pain level, we will take a look at the Silbernagel combined loading program.[64]

We will now present, from our perspective, five of the most glaring issues within the tendinopathy research.

First, there are limited amounts of research pertaining to training programs within scientific literature and, even the ones that are researched have many disparate loading protocols. This is a big problem because one cannot accurately decipher the effectiveness of small modifications on the results of a certain loading program. For instance, only the heavy-slow resistance loading program conforms to a 3x per week frequency when we know the net collagen synthesis is only positive after about 30-36 hours. The overall frequency and set/repetition volume of the Alfredson, Stanish and Curwin, and Silbernagel programs seems to be well tolerated, with good results, for most patients in the case studies. However, we don't know if these programs performed at a 3x per week frequency rather than 2x daily. 1x daily could possibly be more effective with slight changes (higher or lower) in the volume of sets and repetitions to compensate.

From a training perspective, the science of strength and hypertrophy training is far ahead of our current rehabilitation knowledge. Schoenfeld et al did a systematic review and meta-analysis to examine the frequency of training (1-3x per week) for maximization hypertrophy on a volume-matched basis with 2x and 3x per week frequency as superior to 1x per week.[65] Dankel et al found similar results to Schoenfeld, but also noted

Example of Silbernagle Combined Loading Program

PHASE 1: WEEKS 1-2

Goal: start to exercise, gain understanding of their injury and of pain-monitoring model

Patient status: pain and difficulty with all activities, difficulty performing ten 1-legged heel raises

Treatment program: perform exercises every day

- Pain-monitoring model information and advice on exercise activity
- Circulation exercises (moving foot up/down)
- 3x, 10-15 reps: two-legged heel raises standing on the floor
- 3x, 10 reps: one-legged heel raises standing on the floor
- 3x, 10 reps: sitting heel raises
- 3x, 10 reps: eccentric heel raises standing on the floor

PHASE 2: WEEKS 2-5

Goal: start strengthening

Patient status: pain with exercise, morning stiffness, pain when performing heel raises

Treatment program: perform exercises every day

- 3x, 15 reps: two-legged heel raises standing on edge of stair
- 3x, 15 reps: one-legged heel raises standing on edge of stair
- 3x, 15 reps: sitting heel raises
- 3x, 15 reps: eccentric heel raises standing on edge of stair
- 3x, 20 reps: quick-rebounding heel raises

PHASE 3: WEEKS 3-12 (LONGER IF NEEDED)

Goal: heavier strength training, increase or start running and/or jumping activity

Patient status: handled the phase 2 exercise program, no pain distally in tendon insertion, possibly decreased or increased morning stiffness

Treatment program: perform exercises every day and with heavier load 2-3 times/week

- 3x, 15 reps: one-legged heel raises standing on edge of stair with added weight
- 3x, 10 reps: sitting heel raises
- 3x, 15 reps: eccentric heel raises standing on edge of stair with added weight
- 3x, 20 reps: quick-rebounding heel raises
- Plyometric training

PHASE 4: WEEK 12-6 MONTHS (LONGER IF NEEDED)

Patient status: minimal symptoms, morning stiffness not every day, can participate in sports without difficulty

Goal: maintenance exercise, no symptoms

Treatment program: perform exercises 2-3 times/week

- 3x, 15 reps: one-legged heel raises standing on edge of stair with added weight
- 3x, 15 reps: eccentric heel raises standing on edge of stair with added weight
- 3x, 20 reps: quick-rebounding heel raises

that it has yet to be investigated whether or not higher frequencies are more beneficial while understanding that higher frequencies can become more problematic for one to implement.[66] Likewise, McMaster et al has performed a systematic review on the frequency of strength training on a non-volume-matched basis to determine which particular frequency (2x, 3x, 4x per week) is most effective.[67] They concluded, when it comes to non-volume-matching, 3x per week is superior to both 2x and 4x per week.

To our knowledge, no tendinopathy studies have examined any loading programs on a volume-matched or even a non-volume-matched basis. They have only compared the majority of the most common loading programs referenced. Additionally, the high-frequency loading regimens for tendinopathy rehabilitation are in "uncharted territory," as we don't know if the results could be equally sufficient with lower-frequency regimens.

If you are interested in learning more, *Sci-fit* has an excellent overview of the strength and hypertrophy research,[68] and *Stronger by Science* has an excellent overview of the hypertrophy research.[69]

• • •

Second, populations matter significantly. This should be obvious, but it is rarely distinguished in tendinopathy studies while it is more readily distinguished in strength and hypertrophy studies.

A sedentary patient or a patient with overuse injuries due to their occupation represents a significantly different population than an athlete who develops tendinopathy. The workarounds and loading parameters you may use with a sedentary person tend to be completely different than what you would use with athletes. There is very little distinguishing between different populations in the tendinopathy studies. Part of the reason for this is it's hard to get a sufficient number of patients to perform a study within a given population. While this is understandable, it limits the scope of how much the data can be generalized to each population.

The 2009 ACSM guidelines on progression models for resistance training in healthy adults adequately shows the limitations of the current tendinopathy studies.[70] They are able to make recommendations based on different populations, frequencies, and loading parameters including repetition ranges, rest times, velocity, and so on.

For novice (untrained individuals with no Resistance Training (RT) experience or who have not trained for several years) training, it is recommended that loads correspond to a repetition range of an 8-12 repetition maximum (RM). For intermediate (individuals with approximately 6 months of consistent RT experience) to advanced (individuals with years of RT experience) training, it is recommended that individuals use a wider loading range from 1 to 12 RM in a periodized fashion with eventual emphasis on heavy loading (1-6 RM) using 3 to 5-minute rest periods between sets performed at a moderate contraction velocity (1 to 2-second CON; 1 to 2-second ECC). When training at a specific RM load, it is recommended that a 2-10 percent increase in load be applied when the individual can perform the current workload for 1-2 repetitions over the desired number.

The recommendation for training frequency is 2-3 days per week (-1) for novice training, 3-4 days per week (-1) for intermediate training, and 4-5 days per week (-1) for advanced training. Similar program designs are recommended for hypertrophy training with respect to exercise selection and frequency. For loading, it is recommended that loads corresponding to 1-12 RM be used in periodized fashion with emphasis on the 6-12 RM zone using 1 to 2-minute rest periods between sets at a moderate velocity. Higher volume, multiple-set programs are recommended for maximizing hypertrophy. Progression in power training entails two general loading strategies: 1) strength training and 2) use of light loads (0-60 percent of 1 RM for lower body exercises; 30-60 percent of 1 RM for upper body exercises) performed at a fast contraction velocity with 3-5 minutes of rest between sets and 3-5 sets per exercise. It is also recommended that emphasis be placed on multiple-joint exercises, especially those involving the total body. For local muscular endurance training, it is recommended that light to moderate loads (40-60 percent of 1 RM) be performed for high repetitions (>15) using short rest periods (<90 seconds).

The tendinopathy research does not contain anywhere near this level of detail.

• • •

Third, there are other issues to contend with in the studies. The loading programs of many studies do not distinguish between potential stages of tendinopathy, though they will modify for pain. In conjunction with this, many of the studies do not have alternative progression (less or more) for patients that present with tendinopathy who don't respond well or respond exceptionally to the loading programs in a certain stage of irritability. You can see similar phenomena in coaching and personal training. A "beginner program" such as Starting Strength, StrongLifts 5x5, or others may work well for much of the population as a one-size-fits-all program, but a good coach will be able to make adequate adjustments to the training program based on a client's individual needs. In this regard, working around some of the limitations while continuing to help them progress is very similar to rehabilitation.

Some of the factors that are not discussed in these rehabilitation stages that you need to keep in mind are things like risk factors to tendinopathy, technique or form during specific exercises, and even patient compliance. For instance, poor scapular movement patterns or poor technique during exercises can increase stress at the shoulder or elbow, which can contribute to tendinopathy in these areas.

Even some of the authors of these studies are beginning to point out that many of the standard loading programs they researched do not adequately address the associated kinetic chain. A 2016 review by Stanisoplous and Malliaras noted that several other studies indicated hip extensor weakness is prevalent in patellar tendinopathy.[71] In conjunction with the hip extensor weakness, poor lumbopelvic control can alter movement mechanics at the knee due to the gluteal role in controlling internal rotation and external rotation of the knee. Thus, some type of adjunct exercises should probably be recommended for the local area around the injury in conjunction with the main exercises for the tendinopathy.

Beyer et al found similar clinical results between eccentric training and heavy-slow resistance; however, there was more overall patient satisfaction in both the short and long-term (the numbers are only significant in the short term) and in compliance rates.[72] Hence, although some programs may be as effective as others when it comes to differing loading parameters and frequency, there are other factors that should be kept in mind when selecting an appropriate program.

• • •

Fourth, it is important to address deficits, not just within the area of tendinopathy, but also with the associated areas. These include both at the area, as well as proximal and distal kinetic chains:

- Deficits in range of motion.
- Weakness or lack of strength and endurance, especially sport activities or repetitive movements.
- Lack of stability or poor control of movements.
- Pain related alternations resulting in compensatory movement patterns.

One of the big alterations that we have made with our clients to help them return to their sports is a modification of the exercises according to their level of pain and irritability. For example, if a patient is having symptoms of golfer's elbow, distal biceps tendinopathy, or rotator cuff tendinopathy with fixed bar chin-ups or pull-ups, having them perform this exercise on gymnastics rings (where there is free rotation of the hands) can often decrease and/or eliminate their symptoms altogether. The probable reason why this works is that the fixed hand placement of the chin-ups or pull-ups locks the elbows and shoulders into a specific motion which may easily aggravate the tendons at those joints.

The same is true of many exercises where recreational athletes and lifters get tendinopathy, such as squats, bench press, and other exercises where there is a relatively fixed motion at a joint. A modification to dumbbells or unilateral exercises can help mitigate the aggravation without reducing the ability of the client to continue to train. The same is also true of those who have certain occupational hazards leading to repetitive strain injuries (RSI) or tendinopathy.

Exercise modifications also help to reduce the irritability of the tendinopathy so that rehabilitation progresses in a more consistent manner with less possible risk of setbacks that can cause a loss of weeks or even months of dedicated rehabilitation. This is very important knowledge that both healthcare providers and patients should keep in mind in addition to rehabilitation progress.

• • •

Fifth, the aforementioned Malliares review does have some good clinical recommendations despite acknowledging many of the similar limitations already discussed.

> Clinicians should consider eccentric-concentric loading alongside or instead of eccentric loading in Achilles and patellar tendinopathy. Eccentric-concentric loading may be particularly important among patients with marked concentric weakness who may not recover with isolated eccentric loading, due to muscle contraction type specificity. The Silbernagel combined program seems to be an ideal progressive loading program for this patient subgroup. Heavy load training, as in HSR or load maximized eccentric loading, may be more likely to achieve tendon adaptation and may be better suited to some patient groups (e.g. less irritable or degenerative tendon symptoms, high-load demands such as athletes).

> This review has highlighted a dearth of clinical evidence comparing rehabilitation programs in Achilles and patellar tendinopathy. Rather than accepting isolated eccentric loading as the gold standard, studies are needed to investigate how load intensity, time under tension, speed, contraction type and other factors influence clinical and mechanistic outcomes. Potential confounders need to be identified and controlled, and also a change in symptoms, long-term clinical outcomes and recurrence

correlated with change in potential mechanisms. Further, correlated mechanistic outcomes need to be investigated in prospective intervention studies to determine if they are causally linked with improved clinical outcomes. It is important to consider when planning future studies that tendons at different points along the symptomatic reactive-degenerative spectrum may respond very differently to loading interventions.

Generally speaking, the Silbernagel combined loading and heavy-slow resistance programs provide some of the more nuanced programming progressions regarding the progression of tendinopathy rehabilitation as opposed to the Alfredson and Stanish and Curwin.

There are similar nuanced findings in a systematic review in 2018 by Lim et al.[73]

Findings from isometric exercises can be trusted to guide clinical practice (Grade A), whereas eccentric exercises can be trusted to guide clinical practice in most clinical situations (Grade B). It is recommended that HSR exercises be applied carefully to individual clinical circumstances (Grade C) and interpreted with care. Isometric exercises appear to be more effective during competitive seasons for short-term pain relief, whereas HSR or eccentric exercises are more suitable for long-term pain reduction and improvement in knee function.

Overall, it is important for medical practitioners to educate themselves as best as possible to know what variables may play a role in selecting the right loading program. Additionally, medical practitioners should modify the loading programs as necessary based on available patient or client presentation and response to said loading program.

CHAPTER 5

PAIN AND TENDINOPATHY

PAIN SCIENCE

One of the major issues with tendinopathy is pain. As we saw in the 2016 Cook et al model, some cases of tendinopathy involve no pain up until the rupture of the tendon. However, it is more often the case, in acute cases of overuse injuries, that there is pain and discomfort that increases progressively as the tendon is being overused. These cases tend to be present when an athlete or even sedentary individual works through the pain because they don't want to give up their training or task. They think they must push through, and it will eventually go away. These are the cases where you can end up in chronic pain. If an injury is persistently aggravated for several months from the initial onset, chronic pain may be the result. In these chronic pain syndromes, it is possible that the supposedly "injured tissues" are actually healthy, but the patient still experiences pain. Thus, explaining pain from a solely musculoskeletal perspective may do more harm than good.[74]

Let's take a step back for a moment to discuss pain more in depth, as it is a very complex topic.

One of the first models of pain was the *gate control theory*. This theory quickly became outdated, and more models began to replace it. The two primary models are the *neuromatrix theory of pain*[75] and the *biopsychosocial model*,[76] both of which attempt to accurately classify the facts that influence pain.

The *biopsychosocial model of pain* asserts that there are biological, psychological, and social factors that influence pain within the body. These factors affect pain perception.

- Biological Factors: Pain from repetitive stress, injuries or trauma, nerve damage, illnesses, and similar phenomena that affect the body itself.
- Psychological Factors: The effect of emotions and thoughts, mood, attention, [lack of] sleep, [increased] anxiety, depression, fear, [lack of] trust, and other factors that may result in altered behaviors.
- Social Factors: Both biological and psychological inputs with pain can play a role in altering your social activities, relationships, work and occupation, and may lead to more isolation.
- Other Factors: These factors usually are external factors that alter any of the above three areas. Examples include medications, lack of available medical care, financial issues, and so on.

Similarly, the *neuromatrix theory of pain* looks specifically at the various biological and psychological factors to a greater degree. The six general areas, verbatim, are as follows:

- Cognitive Issues: Memories of past experiences, meaning (attributed to past experiences), and anxiety.

- Sensory Issues: The nociceptive (pain) inputs from cutaneous, visceral, and musculature senses.
- Emotional Issues: Limbic system and stress mechanisms. The limbic system regulates threat response in the brain.
- Pain Perception: Sensory, affective, and cognitive dimensions. How our brain interprets pain.
- Actions: Both voluntary and involuntary actions. Smash your knee and you may voluntarily or involuntarily rub it to alleviate some of the pain.
- Stress: The immune system, cortisol, and other stress hormones.

These two models represent factors that are known to contribute to pain. For example, stress, anxiety, and lack of sleep are known to effectively increase pain. Avoiding enjoyable activities also increases pain. Knowing these factors is important because you can take steps to avoid certain behaviors that may increase pain, and you may also adopt certain behaviors—such as deep breathing, meditation, or other relaxation methods—that can help decrease pain.

The book *Explain Pain*, co-authored by David Butler and Lorimer Mosely, discusses how pain is ultimately modulated by the brain and other nervous system structures throughout the body.[77] The book gathers and interprets the modern theories of pain science and attempts to explain it in easy-to-understand language and analogies. They argue that pain acts as an alarm system for the body and sends signals to the brain that something is a threat to the body's health. The brain then prioritizes this incoming alarm signal and attempts to respond with the appropriate level of protective and corrective systems the body uses to optimize healing. This system sometimes appears to behave strangely, or breaks down entirely, for various reasons that are often unknown. Pain can also be amplified by environmental influences like stress, unhealthy habits, and life events.

Tendonitis/tendinopathy is no exception to this system, particularly when pain is experienced chronically (for more than three months). Both the brain and local tissue cells remember the positions or movement patterns that they think may be a threat to the body's health and they are put on high alert, which causes more intense pain. In some cases of acute pain and many cases of chronic pain, there may not be any actual bodily damage that occurs as pain signals are sent; it is the nervous system's warning to protect from a perceived threat. It is quite difficult for the person feeling the pain to tell the difference.

One example would be a software engineer who sits in the same static position in front of a computer, typing. After three hours, he begins to feel pain in his shoulder due to the common "head forward, shoulders rounded" position. This pain is an alarm signaling the body that it needs to begin moving the head and shoulders, as they are in an unfamiliar position the body is not accustomed to. These tissues are under excessive strain that the body cannot handle at this point, hence the alarm of pain signaling the need for movement.

If this software engineer does not change his movement habits and continues his pattern of prolonged sitting, his brain and central nervous system will get more and more involved and begin to amplify the pain signal, moving it higher on the priority list. Now, instead of mild pain after three hours of sitting, it's severe pain after twenty minutes, causing the engineer to seek medical treatment. An MRI is done to the shoulder, showing that nothing is objectively wrong with it. In this case, the pain is not indicating tissue damage, it is a warning signal that is growing louder.

Here is another example that may be more specific to the readers of this book. A long-distance runner begins to experience heel pain after increasing the distance she runs each week while training for a marathon. The repetitive overuse of her Achilles tendon causes an abnormal, non-inflammatory, proliferative response, failed healing, and some microscopic collagen disruption. The runner is told by her doctor that running so much mileage has caused "long-term damage." She is advised to rest and is warned that long-distance running can lead to heel pain and even long-term back pain. She refrains from running for a few weeks, which may allow the tendon to recover from reactive or dysrepair (though not degenerative) tendinopathy, and she is eager to return to training. She starts with shorter distances at first and experiences no pain, but as soon as she attempts to run ten miles, the heel pain returns. Her next run is shorter, but she still feels heel pain and also begins to experience pain in her calf and perhaps her back. However, if imaging were done to her Achilles, it would show no damage. Because of what she was told, her brain is now prioritizing running as a damaging activity and her nervous system is sending abnormal, amplified warning signals even though no damage is taking place.

As physical therapists, we resonate with the theories of pain science laid out in *Explain Pain* and see these types of examples in our patients on a regular basis. We will examine or move a body part for a patient in a way they think should not be done and they will jump or wince as though they are pain. We will ask if they are alright and they will say "yes." Then we will do it again (after asking for permission) and there is no pain or reaction. The brain's expectations are driving pain severity, not actual damage being done to the area.

This concept should be taught to anyone experiencing any type of pain, whether it be tendinopathy or otherwise. We think it is important information to state about the nature of pain in hopes that it will help those who may experience more chronic and confusing symptoms.

PAIN EDUCATION

One of the biggest areas of pain science that is now being explored is pain education, as pain is one of the most misunderstood areas of rehabilitation among most patients and many health professionals. These misconceptions negatively affect the rehabilitation process.

Reviews and studies have shown that pain education regarding the different facets of the biopsychosocial and neuromatrix theories of pain directly reduces pain that is measured before and after pain education. Studies have also shown pain education can reduce disability.[78,79,80] For example, dispelling *fear avoidance* is critical in educating those with pain. Mantras like, "Pain is only in your brain," while somewhat true, do not actually help patients manage their pain. Conversely, this phrasing may lead to more detrimental behavior and increased pain over time. Instead, mantras like, "Hurt doesn't equal harm," "Stay active," and "Return to work as soon as possible" help those with pain avoid developing behaviors that have more detrimental psychological and social impact in the long run.[81]

As *Explain Pain* emphasizes, pain is a protective mechanism and not necessarily a symptom of damage.[82] The body's pathways of pain can be over-sensitized to the point that normal positions or movements can sometimes elicit pain. This is one of the factors that can lead to the development of chronic pain. Thus, "How one makes sense of their pain is an important factor for recovery." Desensitizing the limbic and nervous systems through deep breathing, meditation techniques, and other relaxation techniques may also be useful, along with understanding the pain from a biological, psychological, and social perspective.[83]

A recent Louw et al study called *The efficacy of pain neuroscience education on musculoskeletal pain: A systematic review of the literature* summarizes this quite well.[84]

> Pain is complex, and with well-documented issues such as central sensitization, neuroplasticity, changes in endogenous mechanisms, etc., using pain ratings alone as a measure of improvement seems illogical. Even though evidence supports the reduction of pain over time with the utilization of PNE

(pain neuroscience education), a sudden, total resolution of pain is biologically questionable. The concept of reconceptualizing pain, a cornerstone of PNE, aims to have patients see their pain differently. This implies that even though they still experience pain, they think differently about it, equating it to sensitization of the nervous system versus the health of the tissues. Furthermore, this reconceptualization imparts a message of "despite the pain," it is worthwhile to move, exercise, engage, and continue in daily activities and not necessary to seek additional care for the sensitization (pain). This behavior change is the key to changing any patient's healthcare status, that is, smoking, weight gain, etc.

... in five studies, patients received education-only intervention, none of these studies had any ability to decrease pain ratings, whereas five of the six studies that combined PNE with a physical intervention were able to produce a significant reduction in pain ratings. In line with the definition of PNE and the argument that PNE "biologizes" pain, teaching patients about the biology and physiology of a pain experience would make sense. Education-alone may not be sufficient for change. This is important as many clinicians may be under the impression that PNE is education-only intervention.

This type of education for people with chronic musculoskeletal pain (including tendinopathy) is corroborated by additional studies, especially when paired with physical interventions.[85,86] Pain education *must* be paired with movement-based interventions.

For those who have chronic pain issues, it is important to be aware of the factors that influence pain and recovery. During the rehabilitation process, it is critical to not catastrophize the pain, to not avoid certain activities due to the pain (or only avoid them temporarily if they are aggravating an acute injury), and to not change your lifestyle around the pain. It is often hard for both medical practitioners and patients to find the right balance if they are not educated properly on this topic.

One way we like to explain it to our clients is by telling them to avoid *aggravating* exercises instead of *painful* exercises. Here are some examples of the difference between an aggravating exercise and a painful exercise:

- Some exercises may cause pain, but they improve the performance and function of the injured area(s) after the exercise and/or by the next session. Think about rehabilitation exercises: they may cause pain during a session, but the pain is often the same or decreases over time with subsequent sessions.
- Some exercises may not cause pain, but they make the injury worse over time in terms of both pain and function. We may have to examine an individual's activities, sports, or occupation to see if we can find any patterns of what may be aggravating their condition, such as their habits throughout the day, any potential weaknesses or lack of good movement quality, techniques, or even their attempts at doing self-rehabilitation exercises with improper volume, frequency, loading, or other factors.
- Some exercises may be both painful and aggravating to the point that they cause more pain afterward while decreasing function and performance.

The key to progressing in one's rehabilitation, especially in cases of chronic pain (and sometimes in cases of acute pain), is actively increasing strength, endurance, and stability/control with the movement, with or without pain. Remember, pain is not necessarily indicative of injury or harm. As the rehabilitation process continues, the pain will often go away.

For more detailed information about pain neuroscience education, see Louw et al's *The clinical application of teaching people about pain.*[87]

TENDINOPATHY PAIN

A 2014 review by Rio et al attempted to determine the causes of tendinopathy pain.[88] They explored various factors like tendon matrix changes, neovascularization, tendon cell structure and function changes, cytokines, neuropeptides, and neurotransmitters, metabolites, ion channels, and central pain mediators like the brain and spinal cord.

The molecular biology of tendon in pathological and healthy states highlights many potential contributors to pain, and the search for these needs to extend beyond the tendon. Nociception could occur from cell-cell signaling via ion channels that communicate with an afferent neuron that could transmit, suppress or amplify the nociceptive signal. Nociception may be modulated spinally or above and descending mechanisms may exert nociceptive pressure that manifest locally. Finally, pain could be evoked via non-nociceptive mechanisms through a load detection system, which itself could be disrupted via local or central dysfunction. The question of the pain of tendinopathy, physiological or pathophysiological, remains unanswered; however, there is evidence for both—tendon-based nociceptive contributions and extensive mechanisms within the periphery and the CNS.

Ultimately, they could not pin down any one thing that causes tendinopathy pain. It is likely a combination of many different factors that contribute to this pain.

A 2017 study by Raney et al explored the relationship of pain and dysfunctional development of biceps tendinopathy.[89] Like the Rio et al study, they explore many of the mechanisms of pain, which include: nociceptive pain, peripheral and central neuropathic pain, chronic pain, pain pathways (transduction, transmission, perception, modulation), cell and molecules, tachykinins and receptors, Substance P, CGRP, and alarmins.

They also explore the pros and cons of four of the proposed theories—mechanical theory, vascular theory, apoptosis theory, and neural theory—that could potentially influence pain development in tendinopathy.

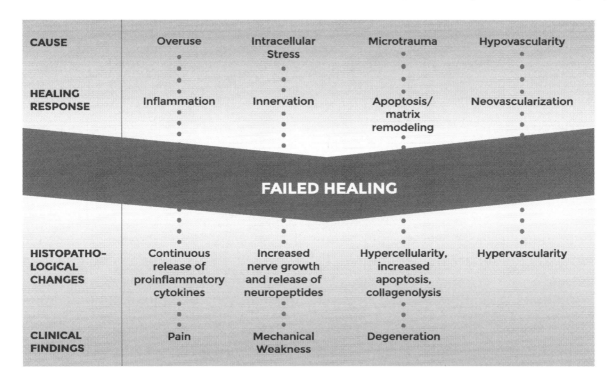

However, like the Rio et al study, the Raney et al study comes to a similar conclusion that more research needs to be done on why there is pain in tendinopathy, as we don't know all the causes and drivers of pain at this time.

Let's switch gears to what we *do* know about how pain interacts with the tendinopathy rehabilitation process.

The Malliares study from the previous section summarized how much pain was allowed in the various loading programs. The Alfredson model allowed pain to be "enough load to achieve up to moderate pain," the Stanish and Curwin models allowed "enough load to be painful in the third set," the Silbernagel model allowed pain to be "acceptable within defined limits," and the heavy-slow resistance model allowed pain to be "acceptable if it was not worse after."

More recent studies like Mascaro et al's systematic graded approach also try to ground their numerical pain scale (in cases non-chronic pain) to show how much pain should be tolerated during exercise, if any.[90]

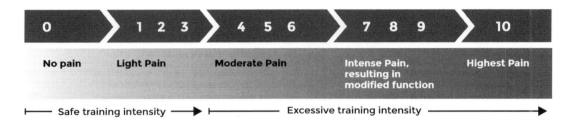

Overall, they tend to suggest sticking to the 0-3 range for pain as a "safe training intensity" because the 4-6 range is excessive training intensity and, often, the 7-10 range is too much pain, resulting in poor technique, compensations, or bad movement patterns.

Although painful exercises may not necessarily be detrimental or cause damage, we personally like to avoid using exercises that may cause pain during the rehabilitation process, if possible. The reason for this is that pain can negatively affect exercise technique due to compensations, even at a low to moderate level. It can also decrease the patients' motivation to get better, and it can negatively affect them psychologically and socially. If there are solid rehabilitation exercises that can be performed and avoid pain, we will use those instead of the ones that elicit pain.

For instance, in some patients who have distal biceps tendinopathy, we may try various types of biceps curl movements (preacher curls, seated arm-on-leg curls, incline curls, standing curls, decline curls, etc.) to see which elicits the least pain, as all are good candidates for distal biceps tendinopathy rehabilitation. Also, we will try the curls with supinated, hammer, and pronated forearm orientations. Many patients have more pain with supinated curls than hammer or pronated curls due to more direct biceps brachii loading as opposed to brachialis and brachioradialis, so we will start with pronated or hammer curls first. We will slowly transition into supinated curls as their load tolerance increases and pain decreases with the two former exercises.

Regardless of the route you take, pain education is necessary. However, if all rehabilitation exercises elicit some pain, it seems that a consensus from the tendinopathy loading protocols is that pain should generally be minimal to absent and should not be worse after the rehabilitation exercises are completed, the day after, or by the next session.

Because there are some instances when working through pain may be detrimental, we tend to recommend that "painful" exercises be performed under the supervision of a rehabilitation professional. For instance, most patients or athletes do not have a good understanding of the types and volume of exercises required in the rehabilitation process. It is often the case that someone trying to utilize painful, but beneficial exercises, on their own may push themselves too far and make their injury worse. Hence, it is important to get professional rehabilitation advice if you have an injury.

Recently, isometric exercises have come to the forefront in tendinopathy research for their ability to reduce pain, especially in in-season athletes. This leads us to the next section of this book.

MANAGING TENDINOPATHY PAIN WITH ISOMETRICS

If the pain is moderate to severe and is limiting or preventing a patient from performing rehabilitation exercises, isometric exercises can be used for pain management.

A few studies have showed isometrics to be effective for pain management. For example, Rio et al examined isometric interventions vs. isotonic interventions in a single-blinded, randomized cross-over study. Their interventions investigated a 70 percent maximum voluntary isometric contraction (MVIC) for 5 sets of 45-second isometrics with 2 minutes of rest compared to 4x8 isotonic exercises at 8-repetition maximum with a 4-second eccentric and 3-second concentric motion.[91] This led to four different results:

- Both resulted in greater pain relief, but the isometric intervention decreased pain significantly more (7.0 ± 2.04 to 0.17 ± 0.41) during a follow-up single leg squat rehabilitation exercise than the isotonic intervention (6.33 ± 2.80 to 3.75 ± 3.28 ($p<0.001$)).
- The isometric intervention decreased cortical inhibition while the isotonic intervention did not. This means that the patients could perform exercises better as cortical inhibition decreases motor drive and the ability to exert strength.
- The isometric intervention decreased pain up to 45 minutes later, but not in the isotonic intervention itself.
- The maximal voluntary isometric contraction increased significantly compared to baseline and the isotonic intervention.

This led to the following conclusion: "Isometric muscle contractions may be used to reduce pain in people with PT without a reduction in muscle strength," especially before rehabilitation exercises that might typically cause pain, such as a single leg squat.

A follow-up study by Rio et al performed on in-season athletes revealed similar findings with a slightly different protocol.[92] This time they used 80 percent MVIC for 5 sets of 45-seconds compared to 4 sets of 8 repetitions at 80 percent, 1 repetition maximum. Their conclusions were similar in that both exercises reduced pain, but the isometric intervention resulted in greater pain relief over a four-week period. Similar studies showed comparative results.[93-94]

Similar options include a study by Pearson et al, which showed that 24 sets of 10 seconds had comparative pain relief as 6 sets of 40 seconds at 85 percent MVIC over a four-week period.[95] This provides an alternative to longer-duration isometrics, which aren't tolerated well in certain populations with tendinopathy.

A systematic review by Lim et al examining isometric, eccentric, and heavy-slow resistance interventions in high-to-moderate quality studies for patellar tendinopathy helped to clarify some of these findings.[96] They found Level A (strong evidence) for isometric interventions, Level B (moderate evidence) for eccentrics in "most clinical situations," and Level C (weak evidence) for heavy-slow resistance, which should be used in individual circumstances with care. Along with this, isometric interventions tended to work well for short-term pain relief, especially with concurrent in-season training where you may not want to reduce as much of the training volume for athletes. However, eccentrics and heavy-slow resistance tended to work best for long-term pain relief and improved function.

Therefore, we tend to suggest using isometrics in three primary scenarios:

- For use in athletes to help decrease pain while maintaining volume of sport-specific activities during competition seasons.
- For pain relief prior to eccentric-concentric or heavy-slow resistance interventions in rehabilitation, especially if they are having difficulty or poor control performing the rehabilitation exercises due to pain.
- Isometrics can be performed multiple times throughout the day to reduce pain, even on non-rehabilitation days.

Although the current isometrics studies are mostly for patellar tendinopathy, they seem to be generally reproducible in other areas of the body. The angle used in multiple studies for the isometric patellar tendinopathy was a 60-degree knee flexion.

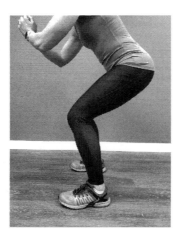

Example of a 60-degree knee flexion. This can also be performed with a leg extension machine.

This would be in the middle of the range of motion for an exercise like a decline board squat or near the end of range of motion for a single leg squat or step down for patellar tendinopathy. Thus, you can likely use the exercises recommended in the next few sections as isometrics for each part of the body by holding the position close to the middle of the range of motion. We are fans of what works best for each individual, so if you find a certain angle that works the best for you in practice for reducing pain then, by all means, use it.

Anywhere in the 70-85 percent 1 repetition maximum MVIC seems to be effective for pain, which according to the National Strength and Conditioning Association (NSCA) training load chart is a weight you can lift for 6-12 repetitions.[97]

The total volume of isometric pain-reduction intervention holds ranges from 3-4 minutes, based on studies that used 5 sets of 45 seconds (3:45 total), 6 sets of 40 seconds (4:00 total), and 24 sets of 10 seconds (4:00 total). We tend to prefer less sets and longer amounts of time, but you can modify accordingly based on what works best for you and/or your patient. We also don't doubt that a possible lower (or even higher) volume of total hold time can be more, less, or as effective for pain relief, but that hasn't been established in scientific literature at this time. You can modify as necessary based on the presentation of the particular tendinopathy based on your best clinical judgement.

CHAPTER 6

TENDINOPATHY PROGRAMMING, PROGRESSION, AND REHABILITATION

The past several chapters have focused on much of the background knowledge for tendinopathy rehabilitation. This chapter will focus specifically on more prescriptive knowledge in order to build a rehabilitation program. There is some overlap between each, but this chapter is more practical in nature.

ORDERING OF REHABILITATION AND PREHABILITATION

One of the basic ways to structure rehabilitation is similar to the way you would structure a training program. This structure is used in Steven Low's book, *Overcoming Gravity*.[98]

1. Warm-Up and Mobility
2. Skill or Technique Work (Handstands, Flips, Gymnastics Tumbling, Breakdancing Work, etc.)
3. Power, [Strength] Isometrics, [Strength] Eccentrics, Regular Strength Work
4. Endurance, Metabolic Conditioning, Tabata Method, Interval Training, Specific Exercises, etc.
5. Prehabilitation, Flexibility Work, Cool Down

The general premise of the warm-up and mobility section is to prepare the body for exercise. This is even more important with an injured area, which can be easily susceptible to reinjury.

The skill and technique work section can be used in rehabilitation to work on proper movement patterns, especially if poor movement patterns have been identified in contributing to the dysfunction or injury. This is where a physical therapist can do well to identify which movements are aggravating your injury to see if there are any dysfunctional or compensatory patterns that may raise your risk of injury or make your condition worse.

The next two sections, which will cover power and strength work and endurance types of exercise, are generally structured in this order since high-power or strength work tends to be more neurologically fatiguing, whereas endurance tends to contain more muscular or cardiovascular taxing exercises. This maximizes the amount of quality work one can perform in a session. This is where a patient will be performing eccentric-concentric or heavy-slow resistance rehabilitation exercises, or more advanced movements, as they progress in rehabilitation.

Finally, prehabilitation, flexibility, and cool-down work is often performed at the end of an exercise session. Isolation work is usually at the very end to work on weak links or to injury-proof the body. Likewise, flexibility work is also performed near the end of a session, as the body will be more fatigued and can more easily relax and stretch more effectively.

This is a general structure that one can use to order rehabilitation sessions with a few modifications.

SAMPLE REHABILITATION SESSION

First, before any rehabilitation work is performed, the irritability stage needs to be determined. If the tendinopathy is highly irritable, it may be made worse by certain types of rehabilitation work, which may need to be removed from your workout. Also, if it is highly irritable, isometric exercises at a minimum may need to be added for pain management, so that any rehabilitation work can be performed with as much pain reduction as possible.

Let's look the ordering of a sample rehabilitation session:

1. Warm-up and Mobility: Mobility and very light stretching, especially if the tendon is stiff to warm up. Heat can be added to help warm up the surrounding tissues if they are exceptionally stiff and painful.
2. Skilled Techniques: Soft tissue work such as massage, manual therapy, or mobilization at a clinician's discretion. Neuromuscular training can be used to focus on good movement patterns.
3. Pain management: Isometrics to reduce pain for the tendon loading program. Heat, and possibly analgesics, can be used as well. If necessary, this can be done prior to a warm-up and skilled techniques.
4. Targeted eccentric-concentric exercises: For golfer's elbow: wrist curls; for tennis elbow: reverse wrist curls; for biceps tendinopathy: biceps curls; for patellar: decline board squats, etc. If a patient is further along in the rehabilitation process, compound exercises and sport-specific movements or occupational tasks can be added.
5. Peripheral strength/endurance or other kinetic chain exercises: This can include strengthening antagonists to make sure there are adequate ratios of strength and the muscles are strengthened proximal and distal to the joint. If there is a lack of control, stability, or weakness above and below the joint(s) where the tendinopathy is located, you can work on that here, too.
6. Flexibility and any follow-up mobility work: Performing mobility work after flexibility work can be sustainable if there is new range of motion created from the flexibility work. Some prefer placing flexibility before strength work, which can also be effective as long as it doesn't interfere with one's strength training.

Various modalities or other interventions can be placed into this schema at one's discretion. For example, extracorporeal shockwave therapy can be done before exercises around points two and three, or on its own.

We now have a solid overview for how to structure rehabilitation sessions. Medical professionals can use this or their own ordering if they find one that is more effective.

PROGRAMMING AND PROGRESSION

Intensity, volume, and frequency make up the main factors that comprise a good progressive loading program for development of strength, endurance, and other attributes as well as proper injury rehabilitation. Let's examine the practical considerations in conjunction with the limited research on the topic.

Intensity and Volume

Intensity and volume are usually intertwined with each other, which is why they are being grouped together here. Intensity determines the repetition range you use during an exercise. Generally speaking, at higher intensities you need to perform more total sets of an exercise to produce a sufficient positive adaptation. In weightlifting, the Prilepin Tables are an example of this. Hypertrophy training is generally performed in the 5-12 repetition range because it produces sufficient intensity and the amount of total volume produces a hypertrophy response.

Exrx.net has a compilation of percentage of 1-repetition maximum at different rep ranges by Brzycki, Baechle, and dos Remedios formatted into a calculator.[99]

Estimated Reps at Percent of 1 Repetition Maximum

Reps:	1	2	3	4	5	6	7	8	9	10	11	12	15
Brzycki	100	95	90	88	86	83	80	78	76	75	72	70	
Baechle	100	95	93	90	87	85	83	80	77	75		67	65
dos Remedios	100	92	90	87	85	82		75		70		65	60

Various loading programs we studied have similar intensities for each exercise. Visnes and Bahr provide a good summary for Alfredson and Stanish and Curwin.[100]

- Alfredson recommends performing two exercises (3 sets of 15 repetitions) at a frequency of twice daily.
- Stanish and Curwin recommends performing one exercise (3 sets of 10 repetitions) at a frequency of once daily.
- The Silbernagel combined loading program begins phase one with four exercises (3 sets of 10-15 repetitions), moves into phase two with five exercises (3 sets of 15-20 repetitions), performs four exercises (3 sets of 15-20 repetitions) in phase three, and closes out phase four with three exercises (3 sets of 15-20 repetitions). The difficulty of each exercise progresses in each phase.
- Heavy-slow resistance begins with three exercises (4 sets of 15 repetitions) and progressively builds toward six exercises.

According to the repetition maximum (RM) percentages, the 10-15 RM range is approximately 60-75 percent 1 RM. This can be used to calculate approximate intensities for isometric exercises in the 70-80 percent range, as well as the loading needed for rehabilitation work.

The relative intensity of the exercises is similar with most programs (that suggest 10-15 repetitions) initially, but there is a significant gap in how much volume is prescribed according to each rehabilitation program:

- Alfredson: 6 total sets per day, 12 total sets every two days, 42 total sets per week.
- Stanish and Curwin: 3 total sets per day, 6 total sets every two days, 21 total sets per week.
- Silbernagel combined: 12 total sets per day (in phase one), 24 total sets every two days, 84 total sets per week.
- Heavy-slow resistance: 6 set average per day, 12 total sets every two days, 42 total sets per week.

Because there is a large disparity from the program volume, ranging from approximately 12, 6, 24, and 12 sets every two days and 42, 21, 84, and 42 sets per week, it is very hard to draw any accurate conclusions. The Silbernagel combined program sets are also a bit misleading since quite a few of the exercise variations are performed at a lower intensity (seated heel raises and standing two leg heel raises) compared to their high-intensity counterparts (standing one leg heel raises and eccentric heel raises performed on the floor).

The Visnes and Bahr study above estimated that the Alfredson and Stanish and Curwin had a patient improvement rate of 50-70 percent over the course of the programs. Habits et al suggests the Alfredson study may provide the best results for mid-portion Achilles tendinopathy.[101] However, the Malliares review suggests that heavy-slow resistance may provide the best results for patellar tendinopathy.[102]

We suspect there is variation in the research because very few studies have protocols that:

- Identify the stage of the tendinopathy (reactive/dysrepair versus degenerative or reactive on degenerative) and the impact that has on the rehabilitation programming.
- Identify the overall irritability or reactivity of the tendinopathy. If it is easily aggravated by loading or progression in loading, then the program may need to be adapted on the fly.
- Identify if the pain the patient is experiencing is acute or chronic and provide accurate and effective pain education.

Therefore, we leave it up to clinician discretion on which eccentric-concentric rehabilitation loading program they want to employ if any and to modify as needed.

Given the variety in the research, we recommend performing 6-12 sets (of 10-15 repetitions per set) every two days for an average of 60-180 repetitions per each two-day rehabilitation session), or a total volume of 21-42 sets per week. However, this is not a hard and fast rule. If a patient is presenting with symptom(s) that are very reactive or irritable, we recommend an initial ramp-up period of a few weeks where one would only perform a few sets of a couple of different exercises.

Frequency

The Alfredson program includes rehabilitation exercises twice a day, while Stanish and Curwin and Silbernagel include daily rehabilitation. Heavy-slow resistance, on the other hand, has rehabilitation 3x per week. There is also a variation within the sets, repetitions, progression, and how much pain is tolerated during each of the exercises.

We generally recommend performing rehabilitation exercises 3x per week, as is suggested in the heavy-slow resistance program, for a few reasons. Patient compliance in performing exercises is much higher when they are only asked to perform them a few times a week, as opposed to every day or even twice a day. Also, as we learned a few chapters prior, different amounts of stress within a rehabilitation program can achieve maximum collagen synthesis rates without the need to perform multiple sessions to obtain enough stimulus on the tendon (though this may not matter since therapeutic exercise results may not necessarily be based on structural changes). Additionally, it's easier to find the correct volume of stress with one session as opposed to having to perform multiple sessions on a tendon that is already irritable or proves to irritate very easily during rehabilitation sessions.

This does not necessarily mean that rehabilitation should only be performed 3x per week with no other exercises. Additional work, such as flexibility exercises, may cause one to respond better to a higher frequency. Likewise, if an athlete or worker is initially having trouble with pain every day, they can perform daily isometrics for the pain if they help to reduce it enough that they can continue in their sport or activity without aggravating their condition. Additionally, different portions of a rehabilitation session can be performed at different frequencies. For instance, concentric-eccentrics can be performed 3-4x per week. The rest of the movements, which include mobility work, soft tissue massage, heat, isometric exercises, and so on can be performed 5-7x per week. If the rest of the peripheral work helps to improve one's quality of movement and makes it feel better overall at a higher frequency, then, by all means, do it.

Given the variety in the research, we recommend starting with 3x per week eccentric-concentric strength training and modifying from there based on how the patient presents and according to the intensity and volume recommendations as needed. The benefits of less frequency per week on improving patient compliance and possible synergy with the collagen synthesis rates and helpfulness with highly irritable tendons makes this a good choice.

Tempo

Tempo is comprised of four different intervals during exercise:

1. Eccentric: The muscle-lengthening phase. In the example of a pushup, this would be the phase where you lower yourself to the ground.
2. Bottom of the Exercise: The amount of time you pause, if any. To use the example of a pushup again, this would be the time you hold at the bottom of the movement.
3. Concentric Phase: The muscle-shortening phase. In a pushup, this would be the phase where you contract your triceps, chest, and shoulders to "push up" to the top.
4. Top of the Exercise: The amount of time you pause, if any. In a pushup, this would be if you pause at the top.

Note: The example above is shown using a pushing exercise. For pulling exercises, the tempo is a 3, 4, 1, 2 sequence. You would begin with the concentric phase, pause at the top, then perform the eccentric phase and pause at the bottom

The tempo of an exercise is often cited in a 4-digit format with eccentric, pause, concentric, pause, such as 10x0. An "X," in this case, means you accelerate *through* the movement, not at a certain time frame. A 3131 tempo would mean you do a 3-second eccentric, followed by a 1-second pause, controlled 3-second concentric, and a 1-second pause at the top.

The tempo for many tendinopathy studies is often not well cited. It usually ranges between 1-5 seconds, if any is mentioned at all. A 2014 study by Bohm et al, in conjunction with their previous experiments, seems to indicate that a tendon strain duration of roughly 3 seconds of loading and relaxation (compared to 1 second loading and relaxation and 12 seconds of loading) is more optimal than shorter and longer loading phases.[103] We already referenced a study in the tendon rehabilitation knowledge chapter that stated that the type of contraction (eccentric or concentric) may not matter. However, there is probably not enough evidence to conclusively say this is the case.

At this juncture, we recommend a 2-3s eccentric and a 1-2s controlled concentric for the initial phases of rehabilitation. The notation for this would be a range of various tempos for the exercises: 3010 or 2010 or 3020 or 2020 tempo. This can be modified based on how a patient is presenting. If they need rest between repetitions or are progressing to a new stage of rehabilitation, a health practitioner may adjust the tempo to make it shorter or faster. If the athletic patient is progressing well, a faster eccentric and concentric portion may be necessary to start preparing them for the explosive and plyometric nature of many sports.

ALTERNATIVE PROTOCOLS

One protocol that I (Steven Low) had been using prior to delving heavily into the tendinopathy research is a higher-repetition protocol. This protocol was developed for the gymnasts, parkour, and climbing athletes I worked with who needed prehabilitation or rehabilitation from their developing injuries in order to transition back to sport. Unfortunately, no official study has been done on this topic, so this is "expert opinion" (Level V evidence).

- 1-2 exercises at 3 sets per exercises.
- 30 to 50 repetitions per set, depending on where you are in progression.
- 2-3s eccentric and 1s concentric, depending on how the tendon is presenting and one's time constraints (3010 or 2010 tempo).
- Stay 3-5 repetitions short of failure, at least to start. This lowers the chance of reinjury.
- Can be performed with pain if the pain does not increase afterward or by the next session and function is improving.

This is a lower-intensity protocol than most of the current research, which typically stays in the 10-20 repetition range for exercises. I initially settled on this for a few reasons. First, an injured area is very easily irritable or aggravated. Hence, a lower intensity and thus higher repetition protocol would potentially be less susceptible to reinjury. An additional benefit of higher repetitions is one can hit volume totals more easily without adding many different exercises. However, the downside to this is many different exercises may hit certain areas more effectively than others, especially if you do different variations of the same exercise.

The progression with this protocol is one of increased repetitions over the different loading protocols, which would typically progress the load (Alfredson), speed of repetitions than the load (Stanish and Curwin), or moving to heavier loads with less repetitions (HSR). It's most similar to the Silbernagel combined program that increases the volume first and then progresses with the exercise:

1. Add 3-5 repetitions (or, more conservatively, 1-2 repetitions) per workout until you hit the 50 range.

2. Then, increase the load or progression of the exercise while lowering the number of repetitions. For example, go from a 5-lb. dumbbell to a 6 or 7-lb. dumbbell and drop the repetitions to the 30 range in order to work back up to 50.

3. Once the tendon function has improved significantly, to the point where heavier loading (10-15 RM) does not aggravate it, begin working in that range. Slowly work toward heavier loads (like 5 RM) if your sport or discipline requires it.

This protocol should be performed three to four times per week, which is similar to HSR and also has a heavier loading phase at the end. However, it begins with a less intense, lower progression rate than most of the tendinopathy protocols mentioned above. This helps to minimize the possibility of reinjury while still getting some rehabilitation loading on the tendons. Overall, I've anecdotally found it has a 60-80 percent success rate.

Here is another interesting anecdote: If high-repetition protocol does not lead to much improvement after a few weeks, it is possible that the other 10-15 repetition protocols will lead to improvement within a few and actually work long-term. This shows us that these protocols are not mutually exclusive.

We can speculate that these different protocols have a slightly different effectiveness rate based on the stage of tendinopathy and how irritable the tendon is (reactive and dysrepair, degenerative, and reactive on degenerative). A tendon in the reactive, or the reactive on degenerative stage, may respond to a higher-repetition protocol initially, as this typically represents a reduction in intensity from typical overuse injuries with high intensity and/or volume. Then, the transition down to 10-15 RM and progressive loading (once the reactive stage(s) have calmed down) can ensure proper loading for the mechanical properties of the tendon to adapt toward healthier norms. Additionally, in degenerative portions of the tendon, with failed healing responses, the lighter load could more readily facilitate maturation of the weaker, type III collagen in the degenerative areas without further aggravating the tendon. This will prepare it for higher loads in the future.

REHABILITATION STAGES

All good training or rehabilitation programs have built-in progressive overload or another form of progression to them, each of which have their pros and cons.

- The progression for Alfredson is to increase the load of the exercises.
- Stanish and Curwin focuses on first increasing the speed of repetitions and then increasing the load.
- The Silbernagel combined loading program focus first on increasing the volume and then progression of the exercise by increasing the load.
- Heavy-slow resistance focuses on moving to less repetitions of heavier loads.

In a patellar tendinopathy article in 2015, Malliares et al suggest a four-phase rehabilitation protocol, which is shown below.[104]

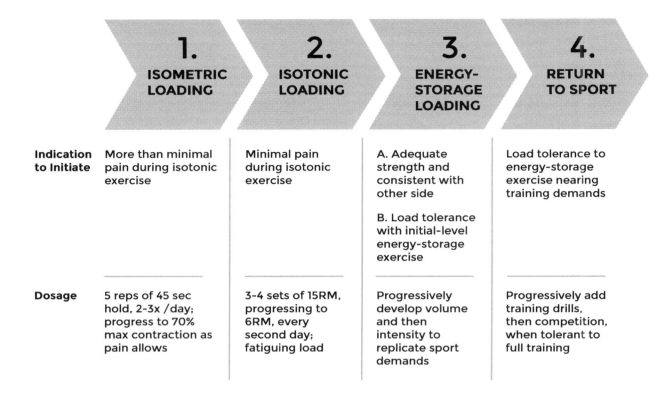

1. ISOMETRIC LOADING	**2.** ISOTONIC LOADING	**3.** ENERGY-STORAGE LOADING	**4.** RETURN TO SPORT
Indication to Initiate More than minimal pain during isotonic exercise	Minimal pain during isotonic exercise	A. Adequate strength and consistent with other side B. Load tolerance with initial-level energy-storage exercise	Load tolerance to energy-storage exercise nearing training demands
Dosage 5 reps of 45 sec hold, 2-3x /day; progress to 70% max contraction as pain allows	3-4 sets of 15RM, progressing to 6RM, every second day; fatiguing load	Progressively develop volume and then intensity to replicate sport demands	Progressively add training drills, then competition, when tolerant to full training

Mascaro et al have a very similar systematic graded approach that focuses on helping athletes return to their sport:[105]

TENDON INJURY

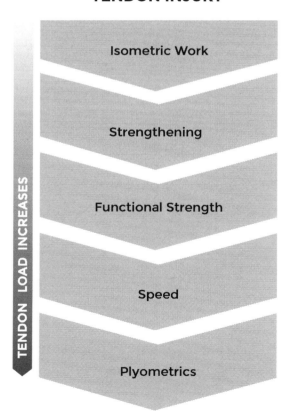

Isometric Work

Strengthening

Functional Strength

Speed

Plyometrics

TENDON LOAD INCREASES

RETURN TO ACTIVITY

Each of these stages are built sequentially to minimize pain and increase strength. They utilize progressive loading to enable rehabilitating athletes to work back toward their sport. This is more obvious to the medical practitioners among us, but often less obvious to the athletes or recreational athletes. Skipping stages of progression can often lead to reinjury because the irritated or degenerative tendon is not ready for the frequency, intensity, or volume of exercise. In fact, the overuse of the tendon with high intensity, volume, or frequency is what caused the injury in the first place.

You may see some individuals progressing more quickly than others because they focus on more advanced progressions too early. This can increase their risk of reinjury, as they could be overloading a tendon that is not ready for heavier weights or faster loading speeds.

Overall, this is a process by which the demands of the rehabilitation program will change over time. The exercises, sets, repetitions, rest times, and other factors will change depending on the state of the tendon and how reactive it is to stress.

Here is a summary/consolidation of both of these programs' recommendations:

1. Reduce Pain and Irritability
2. Improve Strength
3. Improve Functional Strength
4. Increase Power.
5. Develop Stretch-shorten Cycle and Return to Your Sport

We will now cover these five stages in further detail.

Reduce Pain and Irritability

There are several factors to be considered in this rehabilitation stage:

- Clinicians must first distinguish whether the pain is acute or chronic, or whether it is more likely to be one or the other. Proper pain neuroscience education (PNE) must be provided to ensure that the patient has a proper understanding of their pain and is not going to make it worse by catastrophizing it, or thinking that they are doing damage if it is chronic.
- If the tendinopathy is being aggravated by overuse, clinicians should look at a patient's daily life, work, and/or sport in order to recommend which exercises or movements should be removed. They should also recommend removing any exercises that put high tension or compressive loading on the tendon, as this can increase pain and irritability.
- Patients can use isometric exercises to reduce the pain. We recommend 3-4 minutes of total isometric tension, at 70-80 percent MCIV, from 3-24 sets. Typically, sets of 1 minute or 45 seconds are the least tedious. These exercises can be performed multiple times throughout the day as needed.
- Patients can use anti-inflammatory drugs, such as NSAIDs, to reduce pain. Though they may decrease collagen synthesis, you're not introducing exercises for rehabilitation of the tendon at this juncture. Anti-inflammatories may help if there is minimal inflammation (as opposed to none, in many cases) or associated surrounding structural inflammation like paratendonitis, especially in compressed areas like the rotator cuff, infrapatellar area, or Achilles insertion area.
- Other modalities like heat can be helpful to reduce pain. Some evidence has shown that dexamethasone can help calm reactive tendons.
- If there is a reduction in range of motion at the patient's joints, light stretching can be beneficial.

- A skilled medical professional can look for joint weaknesses or compensations above, at, and below the affected area(s), as well as prescribe exercises to begin working on them.

Overall, this phase is designed to eliminate pain and irritability while preparing the tendon for rehabilitation. It is very important to consider the stage of tendinopathy, as this will guide the treatment options in the next phase. Here are the three stages of tendinopathy:

- Reactive/Dysrepair Tendinopathy
- Reactive on Degenerative Tendinopathy
- Degenerative Tendinopathy

If there is reactive on degenerative or degenerative tendinopathy, you must consider that the pain involvement may not respond well to analgesics like NSAIDs, or even isometrics exercises. If the tendinopathy is in the reactive or dysrepair stage, it will typically respond well to a reduction in loading. Additionally, the progression through the next phases of rehabilitation will be rather faster compared to the degenerative cases.

Pain neuroscience education is recommended for both acute and chronic pain. This is done by informing the patient on the nature of both types of pain, although this is most helpful in cases of chronic pain. If you suspect the pain is acute but it is not progressively decreasing as one removes aggravating exercises and progresses in their rehabilitation, it may actually be a case of chronic pain.

Finally, ensure you are also addressing the kinetic chain above and below the area of tendinopathy.

Improve Strength

The goal of this rehabilitation phase is to begin to reintroduce the tendon to loading, typically through isolation exercises that involve eccentric-concentric contractions. This will increase one's tissue load tolerance. Pain will fluctuate in this phase, but should generally decrease unless the pain is chronic. Focus on looking for improvements in tissue strength without reaggravation of the injury.

In this phase, you will also begin to look for compensation patterns or other issues associated with quality of movement. It is typical to see those with tendinopathy pain have decreased control, such as jerky or choppy movements. Thus, it should be a goal to perform each movement in a smooth, controlled manner.

If the tendinopathy is reactive/dysrepair, you can typically combine this rehabilitation stage with the following stage (*improve functional strength*). Substituting aggravating exercises with other strength movements (performed at a lower volume, intensity, and frequency), coupled with isolated eccentric-concentric training is also effective for tendon healing.

You should decrease any sport-specific training to a volume where rehabilitation exercises begin to improve. As a general recommendation, this tends to be about 50 percent (or less) of normal intensity and/or volume while introducing isometric exercises for pain management. It is usually the case that the overuse load has been much higher (30 to 50 percent or more), so reducing the volume of exercises ends up only being a reduction to 65 to 75 percent of one's normal volume.

What is even better is being able to maintain the same intensity and volume of exercise while simply removing any aggravating exercises and replacing them with similar, sport-specific drills that do not increase symptoms and/or decrease function. All of this is at the clinician's discretion since some athletes or sedentary people may do well with only a minor reduction in intensity or volume, while others need a moderate to high reduction.

Reactive on degenerative tendinopathy tends to be highly irritable as you enter this rehabilitation stage. As such, it is important to progress in your exercises slowly. You may need to stick with a consistent volume, intensity, and frequency for two to three sessions (or more) before progressing, as small increases in load volume or the addition of new exercises can easily reaggravate the tendon. You should also be aware that your pain will likely be at a higher level in the beginning of this stage. It should start to calm down but not go away completely. This is because while the "reactive" portion of the pain has subsided, chronic pain from the "degenerative" portion may still be present. Even if this is the case, the overall reduction in pain is a good sign.

Degenerative tendinopathy tends to not be as irritable as reactive on degenerative tendinopathy. At the same time, you will likely experience a reduction in strength and increased atrophy from having been sidelined from your sport or normal routine for an extended period of time. One of the major issues with degenerative tendinopathy is the capacity for chronic pain to develop. Thus, neuroscience pain education is important.

Generally, some simple progressions for improving strength include adding light weights or resistance bands if you are using isolation exercises, which you will find are most common in this phase of rehabilitation. If adding weights, begin with two pounds and progress to three, four, and so forth. If using resistance bands, begin with the easiest and progress with slight increases in difficulty.

Another common progression includes adding an additional set of not-to-failure repetitions, such as going from ten reps to eleven and then twelve and so forth over a period of one to three workouts. The key is using small increases that the tendon can tolerate, so you may want to progress slower if needed. For example, if you are performing three sets of ten repetitions you may add an additional set of one to three repetitions and slowly increase the volume of that fourth set over subsequent workouts.

Here is an overall look at what you should focus on in this phase:

- If pain is an issue, continue isometric exercises. Continue to educate on PNE if you or your patient are having doubts due to a constant level of pain, or if their pain level is not reducing as fast as you think it should.
- Don't progress in your exercises too quickly, especially when coming off reactive or highly irritable tendons. You do not have to progress in every session. If your tendons are responding to the rehabilitation process slowly, it may take two to three sessions to progress.
- Stick with simple progressions for improving strength, such as adding light weights or resistance bands if you are using isolation exercises. You may also utilize additional repetitions, such as increasing repetitions of each exercise from ten to eleven and then twelve over one to three workouts based on your pain tolerance level. Another option is to add an additional set of not-to-failure repetitions. For example, if you're performing three sets of ten repetitions each, you may add a fourth set of one to three repetitions and slowly add volume to that set over subsequent workouts. This can be helpful if you lack the ability for minimal resistance increase.
- Use slow to moderate speed during your repetitions, in both the eccentric and concentric phases. Generally, 2010 or 3010 is a good place to start.
- Aim to slowly increase the progression. This is typically accomplished by load, but repetitions or sets can be a good alternative if it's difficult to increase the load or the reactivity returns due to the load being too high.
- Ensure you are addressing the kinetic chain above and below the area of tendinopathy.

Improve Functional Strength

We tend to not like the word "functional" because it tends to be a buzz word in the fitness world. It refers to transitioning from isolation-type rehabilitation exercises to strength exercises that work fundamental movement patterns applicable for returning to a sport and/or strengthening for a sport.

For example, for lower body tendinopathies, this can mean adding light strengthening exercises that work the lower-body kinetic chain back to your routine (squats, single-leg squats, deadlifts, or other compound exercises). Similarly, for upper body tendinopathies, this can include adding basic exercises like pushups, pull-ups, rows, dips, overhead presses, or similar movements. This may vary depending on your sport of discipline.

There is no rule for when these exercises should be added. In the case of tendinopathy with chronic pain, they may be added rapidly because there may be no actual damage to the tissues that would prevent them from being performed. However, once again, PNE is important to ensure one is not catastrophizing the pain or thinking that it is doing any type of harm.

On the other hand, with reactive tendinopathy or reactive on degenerative tendinopathy, it may be a good idea to wait a week or two after one's rehabilitation exercises have settled their reactivity before beginning to introduce functional strength exercises. This reduces the risk of the reactive tendinopathy returning.

Here is an overall look at what you should focus on in this phase:

- If needed, continue performing isometrics for pain.
- Do not progress too quickly.
- Generally, prior rehabilitation exercises that are easier to perform may be replaced with other, more effective exercises if it is deemed beneficial.
- When one adds compound exercises, they should pay close attention to compensations and application to strengthening the kinetic chain.
- Slowly add these functional exercises as volume. If the volume seems to be too much, one may reduce the isolation exercises in favor of some compound movements. For instance, going with one to two sets of isolation exercises after the compound movements are added.

In the course of normal rehabilitation, the tendon may "flare up," either during the session, after the session, or the next day with a reaction of increased pain, tenderness, and soreness. This is a normal part of the rehabilitation process, as things do not always progress smoothly when you're dealing with an injury. A clinician should examine the rehabilitation program to see if you should stay the course or modify based on how you are presenting. Sometimes, it is best to stay the course, as flare-ups of symptoms can happen regardless of an effective loading scheme, and sometimes you modify. Remember, the goal is increased load tolerance, strength, and function. Basing a rehabilitation program off symptoms is often ineffective and haphazard. It's easy to fall into this trap.

Increase Power

By now, you should have a good idea of how the tendinopathy has responded regarding the reactivity/decreasing pain, improving strength, and improving functional strength phases of rehabilitation. Bear in mind, if the tendinopathy is easily aggravated, you should take it slow and not be in a hurry to progress. On the flip side, if you are progressing well you should focus on consistent improvement that, once again, does not occur too quickly.

As pain decreases (or remains the same) and you continue to improve in both strength and functional exercises, there will usually be a transition period of the functional strength exercises into power by decreasing the eccentric and concentric times gradually until you are performing the repetitions in a more explosive manner.

This is a very straightforward phase, but it is very easy to overdo it. That is why we suggest slowly phasing in exercises that are performed in a more explosive manner. For instance, instead of trying to increase the tempo of several exercises at the same time, focus on one at a time and track both pain and function post-rehabilitation, as well as the next day's function and any symptoms. This will provide gradual progression instead and will aid in avoiding overwhelming the tendon.

Try to avoid exercises that begin with compressing the tendon, such as very deep heel raises and similar power exercises. We recommend you begin by primarily focusing on the muscles at the mid-range as opposed to end-range, as there are usually more compressive loading forces at the joint and these areas tend to be easily aggravated. Slowly progress the power exercises into a larger range of motion and more compressive loading positions if they respond well. For instance, if a climber has golfer's or tennis elbow, the positions that can aggravate it the most tend to be the bottom or top of a pull-up. Therefore, developing power with pull-ups should first be done in a limited range, such as starting with your arms slightly bent and not going up to a full lock-off first. If this responds well for a week or two, you can transition into a more powerful pull-up movement that utilizes your full range of motion.

If you're working with more sedentary patients or active patients who are getting tendinopathy from their work, this phase and the next may not be necessary depending on the activity or task. Instead, more activity or task related activities should be introduced again with emphasis on good movement patterns and strategies to avoid overloading the tendon when resuming full time activity.

Here is an overall look at what you should focus on in this phase:

- Begin with mid-range power work before moving toward end-range work in order to avoid placing compressive loads on the tendon.
- Continue to track your pain and function after your workout, as well as the next day, in order to ensure you aren't progressing too quickly. If the tendon starts to get irritated, have a plan to back off.
- If power is not needed, such as in some sedentary patients or active workers, begin to introduce task-related activities in conjunction with strategies to avoid overuse.
- Make sure you are addressing the kinetic chain above and below the area of tendinopathy.

Develop Stretch-shorten Cycle and Return to Your Sport

The stretch-shorten cycle is the eccentric-concentric rebound motion often termed *plyometrics*, which is typically used in almost every sport that requires sprinting or jumping. Now that you have gradually and gently transitioned your exercises into the power phase, you can begin utilizing them in the context of your sport or discipline. The same concepts from the previous section apply here as well: begin mid-range instead of jumping in to full compressive loading. You can build up the volume and progressions over time.

If your medical practitioner is not as familiar with these exercises, you may want to seek more specialized care, such as a sports doctor or physical therapist. You may also find it beneficial to consult an athletic trainer, coach, CSCS, or other professional with specialized knowledge in order to seek advice on a method of progression for reintroducing exercises to your athletic regimen.

From our experience, most laypeople and athletes who have not trained any type of explosive or plyometric regimens jump into them far too quickly. Depth drops or rebounds tend to be performed with a height that is way too high, and too many repetitions are attempted. Start with a very small amount and don't go to failure. Increase the volume slowly, over time, and add in faster sport-specific movements that increase in speed as the volume increases.

CONTINUING YOUR SPORT DURING REHABILITATION

Many athletes ask, "Should I continue my sport while I am undergoing rehabilitation?"

The short answer is "yes," but you must do it properly.

When your average recreational athlete gets injured during training they usually take a week or two of total rest. If the injury persists, they may even take off for a longer period of time lasting a few months or more depending on the severity of the injury. However, this is generally a mistake. You don't want to totally cease activity for more than a week or two because it doesn't really provide any benefit and it can cause you to lose good habits, leading to atrophy and loss of other adaptive changes. Some athletes have even inadvertently gained weight because they failed to change their nutrition habits after "resting."

Instead of total rest, you want to rehabilitate the part(s) in question (with appropriate medical diagnosis and treatment plans), while still maintaining the habits and benefits of your sport as much as you are able.

The severity of the tendinopathy plays a big role in how soon one can return to their sport. Most athletes who have reactive tendinopathy with low irritability can simply reduce the amount of offending sport-specific movements and do rehabilitation work on the side. The length of rehabilitation can be as short as a few weeks if no setbacks occur, with activity slowing ramping up as the body can handle it. For instance, if an athlete was running for ten hours per week, it would not be wise to drop down to zero activity. Instead, they can simply cut their volume roughly in half (say, four or five hours per week). If the tendinopathy gets worse, the volume should be dropped. However, it can be increased if consistent improvement is seen without compensations. You should also experience a decrease in pain and improved strength and function.

Because it can be difficult to estimate how much activity should be reduced and which specific exercises are aggravating the tendinopathy—especially in sports that aren't as uniform as running—it is good to err on the conservative side. A 40 to 50 percent decrease in volume is typical, but it can range from anywhere between zero to 95 percent. Some athletes can get away with solely removing aggravating exercises from their routine (if it was one specific movement, such as with rock climbing or gymnastics) and continuing all other movements and exercises. Other types of athletes may have to significantly decrease their volume—even down to almost nothing—for a few days or a week in order to see improvement, especially if the tendon is extremely reactive. Even if you are barely doing anything, it is almost always better to attempt some form of exercise than to completely rest. Generally, you should always start with less so you won't re-injure or aggravate the tendon. You can then slowly add more volume and intensity, typically less than 10 percent each week. A good rule of thumb is to focus on non-painful sports activities.

However, everyone will respond to rehabilitation differently, so make sure you are consulting the appropriate medical professionals throughout this process to help guide you in load and pain management. If you don't know who to look for, our general recommendations are doctors, physical therapists, trainers and those who are used to working with athletes. You may want to do some research and see who local sports teams or universities use for athlete care.

Here is an overall look at what you should focus on:

- With any injury, consult with the *appropriate* medical professional. You should make an appointment right away, as there is often a lag time of a couple weeks before you can set an appointment and you will want to get in as quickly as possible for moderate to severe injuries. If it's a minor injury that "heals" itself and you don't want professional help, you can always cancel the appointment. However, even in these cases we would recommend that you still get yourself checked out.
- Generally, you can continue in your training regimen—at least with the movements that are away from the injured areas. For example, if you are dealing with golfer's elbow, continue all lower body and core work. You can typically also continue with exercises around the injury if they do not further aggravate it and increase pain.

PREVENTING INJURY AND REINJURY

What are some measurable and scientific ways to prevent injuries and especially reinjury? This is always a major question for health professionals, coaches, and athletes and occupational workers as they are coming back from an injury. We will now investigate some of the objective measures coming out of the scientific literature that everyone can use to help prevent injury and reinjury.

Acute:Chronic workload ratio (including rate of perceived exertion)

Recently, there has been research on what is called *acute:chronic workload ratio* (ACWR) and the risk of injury in sports. A few analyses were performed earlier, but the one that first brought ACWR to prominence was performed by Gabbett in 2016.[106]

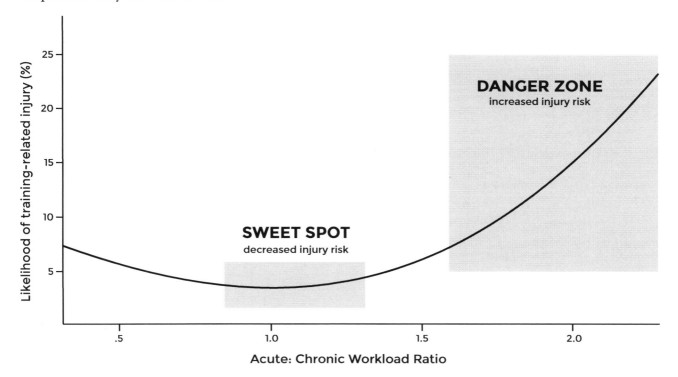

The area where the chance of injury decreases the most is the 0.8 to 1.3 zone of ACWR. Here is their analysis of the chart:

Is there a benefit in modelling the training–injury relationship using a combination of both acute and chronic training loads? Acute training loads can be as short as one session, but in team sports, one week of training appears to be a logical and convenient unit. Chronic training loads represent the rolling average of the most recent three to six weeks of training. In this respect, chronic training loads are analogous to a state of 'fitness' and acute training loads are analogous to a state of 'fatigue.'

Comparing the acute training load to the chronic training load as a ratio provides an index of athlete preparedness. If the acute training load is low (i.e., the athlete is experiencing minimal 'fatigue') and the rolling average chronic training load is high (i.e., the athlete has developed 'fitness'), then the athlete will be in a well-prepared state. The ratio of acute:chronic workload will be around one or less. Conversely, if the acute load is high (i.e., training loads have been rapidly increased resulting in 'fatigue') and the rolling average chronic training load is low (i.e., the athlete has performed inadequate training to develop 'fitness'), then the athlete will be in a fatigued state. In this case the ratio of the acute:chronic workload will exceed one. The use of the acute:chronic workload ratio emphasizes both the positive and negative consequences of training. More importantly, this ratio considers the training load that the athlete has performed relative to the training load that he or she has been prepared for.

Gabbett makes it clear that extrapolating to other sports may not work so well, but were able to find similar results existing between (Australian) cricket, rugby, and soccer for both contact and non-contact injuries in each of the sports. Another important finding is that high chronic workload with a lower ACWR was generally effective at preventing injury. This is likely because the athlete was adapted to the volume and intensity of the exercise. Therefore, a high volume and intensity is not necessarily conducive to injury but a high relative dose. In other words, a high workload is not harmful but rather *too much, too soon*. This was confirmed in another study, and they also demonstrated that you can manipulate volume if there is a short period of recovery between matches/games to decrease injury risk.[107] Hulin and Gabbett nearly replicated their results by finding a similar 0.85 to 1.35 ACWR was the best predictive of decreasing the rate of injuries.[108]

To calculate ACWR, take a one-week workload versus a three to six-week rolling average of the athlete's internal and external workloads and compute it into numbers. External workloads are things like high-speed sporting activities or high mileage. High internal workloads were calculated on the *rate of perceived exertion* (RPE) scale for each session, though that study has not been replicated. If there is a very high increase in internal stress or external activity compared to one's rolling average, there may be a higher risk of injury.

Another study found that *exponential weighted moving averages* (EWMA) may be more sensitive to injury than traditional ACWR with rolling averages.[109] What this means is that more weight is given to recent workouts than a rolling average. Therefore, if the progression is too fast it would predict injury better than a rolling average of the past three to six months. For most people, this is more difficult to calculate, so it might not be feasible option. The key point to remember is *too much, too soon* is not good.

Since these initial studies have been performed, there have been more studies on high-level college and professional athletes, including English soccer players,[110, 111] professional men's basketball,[112] and collegiate American football.[113] Two elite European soccer teams found a 1.0-1.25 ratio helped prevent injury.[114]

If you are not a professional athlete and don't play any of the sports listed above, take this with a grain of salt. There does seem to be a correlation across most sports, but the verdict is still out on how *much* of a correlation. In any sport, there is validity to the notion that progressing too quickly increases your chance of injury.

Heart Rate Variability

Heart rate variability (HRV) has become popular over the last decade for tracking sports performance, as it is helpful to know when to train harder or easier (if you are experiencing fatigue). HRV is a measure of autonomic nervous system function.[115]

Here is a basic example. In the absence of stress, there is high variability between each heartbeat interval. An athlete's 60-beats-per-minute resting heart rate may have 0.9-1.1 seconds (1±0.1s) between each heartbeat. However, when their body undergoes stress, especially chronic stress, the variability decreases and trends toward 1.0 beats per minute (1±0s) at resting heart rate. The variability between the beats decreases from 0.1 seconds to 0 seconds (e.g. high HRV toward low HRV). It may even trend upward in resting heart rate due to the stress. Tracking heart rate when the body is under low HRV will let one know that their workouts have placed a high amount of stress on their body. This lets the athlete know to dial back on their training intensity, volume, or frequency so they can better recover.

In terms of performance, there were similar links between ACWR and HRV. NCAA Division 1 collegiate soccer players had a high correlation of acute:chronic workload ratio based on session time and low HRV and were recommended to help coaches adjust training sessions.[116]

Although there is a growing amount of scientific literature on using HRV for performance and many sports teams are doing this, there isn't much that covers rates of injury. That being said, what research is there is promising. A small study on CrossFit athletes profiling both acute:chronic workload ratio and HRV showed that at high ACWR and low HRV there was increases in susceptibility to reporting an overuse injury the following week.[117] A similar study looked at HRV, blood pressure, and baroreflex sensitivity in track and field athletes.[118] A prospective study using NeuroPlus biofeedback in conjunction with physiological measurements like HRV was able to reduce both injuries and missed training days in elite soccer players.[119] There may even be a link between HRV via sympathetic and parasympathetic drive in swimmers and predicting illness in certain body positions (supine, and supine to standing/orthostatic position) due to the nature of how the heart compensates for beating while laying down and standing up from laying down.[120]

We personally have not seen any healthcare practitioners use these concepts during rehabilitation, but they could be implemented in one's rehabilitation progression. ACWR is a very good indicator that will help one know not to progress in their rehabilitation exercises too quickly if they can track the overall volume, load, and frequency both quickly and effectively.

CHAPTER 7

TENDINOPATHY EXERCISES

In this chapter, we will discuss exercises that can be used to help overcome tendinopathy. Many of these exercises are already well known to most healthcare professionals. We are providing at least one, but usually two or more specific rehabilitation exercises for each tendon. Some patients will find that one particular exercise aggravates their tendinopathy while a different exercise for the same tendon will be fine or even effective. Some exercises are also more advanced progressions than others. For example, some of the rotator cuff exercises place the shoulder at a greater position of instability than others, making them more advanced variations.

When moving from the "improving strength" to "improving functional strength" stage of rehabilitation, there will be a transition into basic compound movements. As mentioned previously, the basic upper-body exercises that tend to be effective are pushups, pull-ups, rows, dips, or overhead press. You can also perform easier movements with barbells if bodyweight exercises are too much. You can also scale these exercises as needed, such as performing wall pushups, incline pushups, or stair pushups if regular pushups are too difficult. Likewise, lower body squats, deadlifts, or other basic barbell or bodyweight exercises can work effectively. The exercises can vary depending on the level of strength needed to return to work or a sport. For this reason, we didn't include many other basic compound exercises beyond the isolation exercises for the tendinopathies, even though they have a place in a good rehabilitation program. Consult your medical professional, especially when you are transitioning from isolation and compound exercises back to your sport.

Most times, tendinopathy affects only one limb. We recommend completing each exercise with both limbs because it allows you to see the difference in range of motion, stability/control, endurance, and strength compared to the healthy limb. These comparisons are useful for determining the degree of impairment. Also, only training one side can lead to imbalances near the end of rehabilitation. For example, if you only train the side affected by tendinopathy it may actually end up stronger than the unaffected side.

Begin with the affected side and follow up with the unaffected side. This will ensure that you match the intensity and volume of the exercise with your stronger side. If you begin with the unaffected side, you may try to match it with the injured side. This can lead to unnecessary strain and potential reinjury, especially among those who are highly competitive.

Some of these exercises can be performed with both arms at once, such as with a barbell, two dumbbells, or a two-handed pulley system. It is generally best, especially early on in the rehabilitation process, to focus on isolating the affected limb and following up with sets from the unaffected limb. As you improve, you can perform both together.

There may be times when a single-limb exercise is too difficult to perform with your affected limb. In these instances (such as with single-leg calf raises for Achilles tendinopathy), assisting with the unaffected leg is your best bet to ensure you do not progress too quickly and aggravate the tendinopathy. As you improve, you may be able to remove this assistance.

Authors' Note: Some of these exercises are found in various studies, while we have used others with our clients. These are not the only exercises that can be used effectively for rehabilitation, so don't feel limited to what you find in this chapter.

You can progress in these exercises by using small dumbbells, bands, or other training implements. Most of the exercises pictured are shown without weights.

ROTATOR CUFF

Both the supraspinatus and infraspinatus/teres minor are the most common tendons to develop tendinopathy. If you are rehabilitating rotator cuff tendinopathy, we typically recommend you perform exercises for both. There is usually subacromial bursa involvement (which makes NSAIDs that decrease inflammation and swelling to the area more effective than they are at treating tendinopathy in other areas). Additionally, because scapular movement and mechanics influence shoulder movement so greatly, you can significantly reduce shoulder pain through scapular strengthening and technique. This is true with tendinopathy, as well as other shoulder injuries.

Exercises for the Supraspinatus Tendon

Sidelying Empty Can

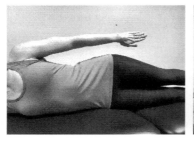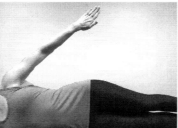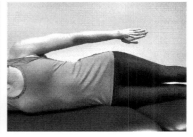

Begin by lying down on a sturdy bench, on your non-affected side. Your affected arm should be on top. Rotate your arm so your thumb is pointed toward your side. Raise your arm to a 45-degree angle, away from your side. Slowly lower your arm using the appropriate eccentric time.

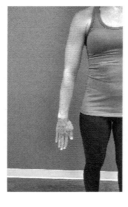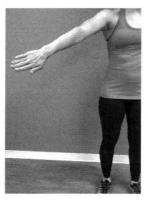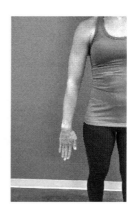

Standing Scaption Raise with Thumb Down

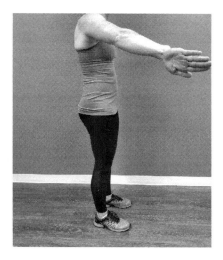

Alternate Angle of the Top of the Standing Scaption

Begin in a standing position, with your arm by your side. Rotate your arm so that your thumb is pointed toward your side. Raise your arm in the scaption plane (between a front raise and side raise; see above for example) with your pinky finger leading the way. Continue raising your arm until it reaches a 65 to 70-degree angle away from your body while remaining below shoulder-height. Slowly lower your arm using the appropriate eccentric time.

This exercise can aggravate the shoulder, so be careful. If you have any issues, you may need to substitute it with another movement.

Scaption plane example: Your right shoulder is affected. If 12:00 is in front of you and 3:00 is your side, you want to raise your arm to approximately 1:30. This is what we mean by the middle position between a front raise and a side raise; it should be roughly 45 degrees between each.

Exercises for the Infraspinatus Tendon

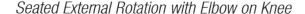

Seated External Rotation with Elbow on Knee

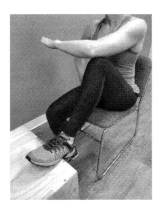
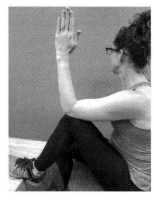
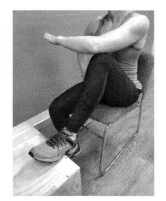

Begin by sitting down on a bench or chair. Put your foot up, so the knee on your affected leg is in a bent position about a foot from your shoulder. Your knee should be several inches below shoulder-height. Place the elbow of your affected shoulder onto your knee. Your elbow should be at a 90-degree angle with your hand pointed up. Slowly allow your hand to rotate inward using the appropriate eccentric time. Pause the motion when your hand reaches or is slightly below elbow-height. Slowly rotate your hand back to the starting position to complete the repetition.

Cuban Press

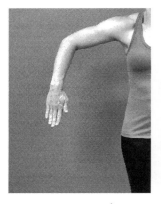 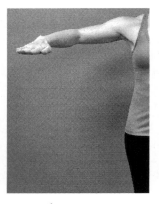 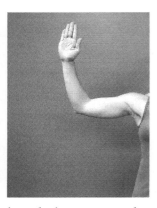 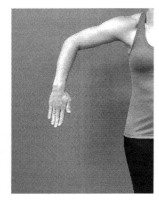

Begin in a standing position, with your arms out to the side, bent at a 90-degree angle, and pointed downward. Keep your elbows still and maintain the position as you slowly rotate your hands forward. As your hands rise, continue to rotate them upward until they reach a U-position where they are pointed upward. Next, slowly allow your arms to rotate downward, back to the starting position, using the appropriate eccentric time.

The external rotation portion of the Cuban press is generally considered a more advanced exercise for external rotation because your shoulder is abducted (raised 90 degrees out to the side) and externally rotated (90 degrees with your arm pointed toward the ceiling at the top position). This 90-90 abduction and external rotation position is one of the most unstable for the shoulder, so if you experience any instability or other issues with subluxation or dislocation it is not wise to start your rehabilitation with this exercise. This is especially important with tendinopathy, as there tends to be decreased motor control and function due to pain and instability.

Exercises for the Teres Minor Tendon

Sidelying External Rotation

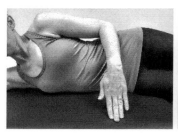 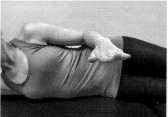 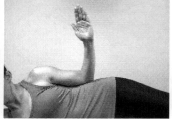 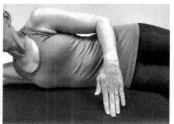

Begin by lying down on a sturdy bench, on your non-affected side. Your affected arm should be on top, against your side, with your elbow bent at a 90-degree angle and hand near your stomach area. From here, rotate your hand upward while your arm remains by your side. Continue to rotate your arm upward until it is above your body. You should either go through your full range of motion or stop just short of discomfort. Next, slowly lower your hand down using the appropriate eccentric time. Ensure that only hand rotation occurs during this movement and your arm remains at your side for the duration of the exercise.

Standing External Rotation with Band or Pulley

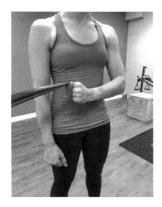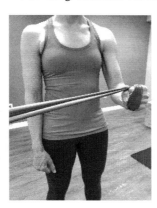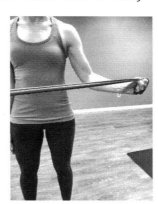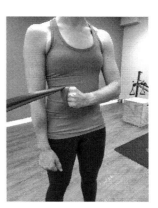

This exercise can be performed with a Thera-Band or pulley system at a gym. Begin in a standing position, with your arm next to your side, hand against your stomach, and elbow bent at a 90-degree angle. Grab the band/pulley so you are facing it at a perpendicular angle and it is parallel with your forearm. Rotate your hand outward, away from your body, in a controlled manner while keeping your arm by your side for the duration of the exercise. You should either go through your full range of motion or stop just short of discomfort. Slowly allow your hand to rotate inward, toward your body, using the appropriate eccentric time.

A pair of gymnastics rings can be particularly helpful as you are resuming upper-body strengthening exercises like pull-ups or chin-ups. This is because the rings allow for free rotation, enabling your wrists, elbows, and shoulders to avoid getting stuck in a particular movement pattern that can aggravate upper-body tendinopathies like golfer's elbow, tennis elbow, biceps, and rotator cuff tendinopathies.

It can be tricky to hit the specific area of the tendon with the infraspinatus and teres minor. If these exercises are not effective, it can be helpful to lie on your side, thus moving your arm up into greater flexion and allowing gravity to assist with external rotation.

GOLFER'S ELBOW (MEDIAL EPICONDYLE) AND ANTERIOR WRIST

We have seen quite a few nuances with golfer's elbow. This is because the common flexor tendon is the origin of several different muscles: the flexor carpi ulnaris, palmaris longus, flexor carpi radialis, pronator teres, and flexor digitorum superficialis. Since the reactive, reactive on degenerative, or degenerative portions of the tendon can be in *any* area of the common flexor tendon, exercises targeting a specific muscle can lead to better strength and load tolerance than other, more general, exercises.

For instance, if traditional eccentric-concentric wrist curls have not helped the tendinopathy in past rehabilitation sessions, it's possible that different, more specific exercises can help. If the area of the pain is more superficial and lateral on the common flexor tendon (along the pronator teres area) then pronation/supination eccentric concentrics may be more effective. Similarly, if the area of pain is deeper on the common flexor tendon, more specific exercises like finger curls (with a dumbbell) or resisted finger pushing up and down against the ground can be more effective.

Here are the three primary themes we have seen:

- Wrist flexion golfer's elbow (flexor carpi radialis/ulnaris-based)—This is typically resolved with wrist curl eccentric-concentrics and pronation/supination secondary work.
- Pronation/supination golfer's elbow (pronator teres-based)—This is typically resolved with pronation/supination as a primary exercise and wrist curl eccentric-concentrics as a secondary exercise.
- Finger flexor golfer's elbow (flexor digitorum superficialis (FDS) based)—This is typically resolved with finger curl-type exercises or eccentrics-concentrics that involve pushing your fingers into the ground to raise up your palm and then lowering slowly. Both hit the FDS with eccentric-concentric and pronation/supination. If needed, wrist curl eccentric-concentrics can be used as supplementary exercises.

In our experience, athletes in gymnastics, climbing, calisthenics, and those who do significant amounts of pullups often get a pronator teres or flexor digitorum-based area of reactive or degenerative tendinopathy. Thus, rehabilitation exercises should place a focused emphasis on loading schemes toward those areas of the tendon, if it can be tolerated. If not, begin with exercises that de-emphasize those areas of the tendon. As the tendon begins to increase in load tolerance, slowly introduce the exercises that target the areas you were previously unable to tolerate. This is similar to the biceps curls example: Begin with pronated or hammer curls and slowly introduce supinated curls (if supinated curls are not well tolerated at first).

We will cover the most common exercises, but if they prove to be ineffective it could be helpful to explore some of these themes further.

You can progress in these exercises by using small dumbbells, bands, or other training implements. Most of the exercises pictured are shown without weights. Additionally, depending on where the reactive or degenerative portion of the tendon lies, your arm can either be straightened or bent further in order to create a bias toward the affected area(s).

Wrist Curl

This exercise can be performed in a seated or standing position. The seated variation is most often preferred because it allows you to stabilize your forearm. However, the standing variation is often better if the seated version aggravates your tendinopathy or fails to work after a few weeks.

For the seated variation, sit in a chair and face parallel to a table. Next, bend your elbow to a 90-degree angle and place your forearm on the table so that the wrist of your affected arm hangs just barely off the edge of the table. Your palm should be face up and your wrist relaxed. From here, raise your wrist toward your body (against gravity) through your full range of motion. Slowly lower your wrist using the appropriate eccentric time.

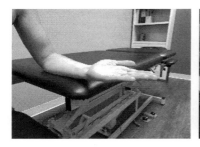 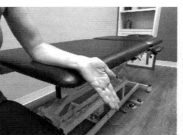 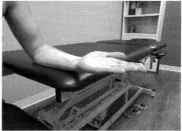

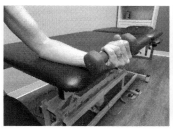 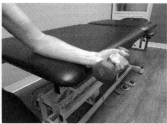 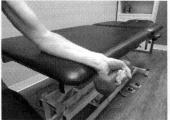 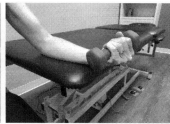

For the standing variation, stand with your arms by your side and your palms facing forward. Curl your hand forward as far as your range of motion allows. Then, slowly lower your wrist using the appropriate eccentric time.

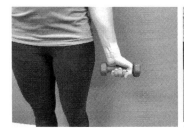 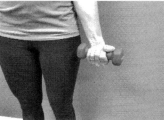 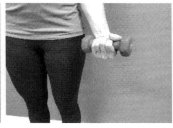 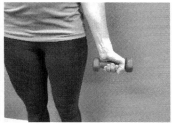

Alternatively, this exercise can be performed with your palms facing backward. You will curl your wrist backward but otherwise perform the exercise in the same manner. The standing variation can be performed with dumbbells or with a barbell. If you are using a barbell, the bar will generally be in front of you for the palms-forward variation and behind you for the palms-backward variation.

Pronation/Supination

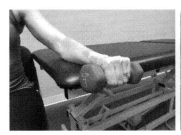 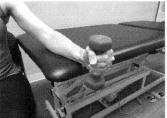 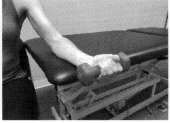 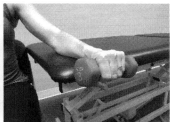

Sit in a chair and face parallel to a table with a dumbbell or, alternatively, the head of a hammer in your hand. Bend the elbow of your affected arm to a 90-degree angle and rest your forearm so your wrist is just barely off the edge of the table. Start with your palm face down and your wrist in line with your forearm and slowly rotate your forearm so the dumbbell rotates from one side to the other (180 degrees) using the appropriate eccentric time when lowering it. Rotate back to the starting position in a controlled manner.

This exercise should be performed in conjunction with wrist curls because the pronator teres muscle has a common tendon origin on the common flexor tendon. This exercise typically helps significantly if there is specific discomfort, tenderness, or pain on the lateral portion of the common flexor tendon, but we have found it's also a solid rehabilitation exercise overall.

As mentioned previously, a pair of gymnastics rings can be particularly helpful as you are resuming upper-body strengthening exercises like pull-ups or chin-ups.

Finger Curls / Finger Rolls (for FDS-based Tendinopathy)

We didn't include photos since these movements are difficult to show in photo form. However, here are two different videos of exercises that can be used to emphasize the FDS: https://www.youtube.com/watch?v=TiXGR4p1dwY and https://www.youtube.com/watch?v=O8_-Ynpyl4g.

TENNIS ELBOW (LATERAL EPICONDYLE) AND POSTERIOR WRIST

There are several differential diagnoses in the lateral epicondyle region that can mask themselves as tennis elbow, so one must ensure that the clinical symptoms are not actually another issue. Both tennis and golfer's elbow are easily misdiagnosed.

Reverse Wrist Curl

This exercise can be performed in a seated or standing position. The seated variation is most often preferred because it allows you to stabilize your forearm. However, the standing variation is often better if the seated version aggravates your tendinopathy or fails to work after a few weeks.

For the seated variation, sit in a chair and face parallel to a table. Bend the elbow of your affected arm to a 90-degree angle and rest your forearm so your wrist is just barely off the edge of the table. Start with your palm face down and your wrist relaxed, in line with your forearm, and begin to raise it up (against gravity) to the end of your current range of motion. Slowly lower it down using the appropriate eccentric time.

If your wrist responds well, you can lower it past the parallel point (not seen in the images below) to work your full range of motion. This is where you will eventually want to be.

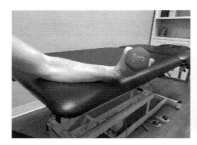 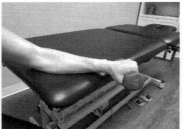 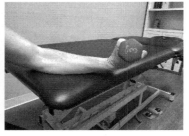

For the standing variation, stand with your arms by your side and your palms facing backward. Next, extend your hand forward as far as your range of motion allows. Slowly lower it using the appropriate eccentric time. If you are using a barbell, the bar will be in front of you for the palms-facing-backward variation and behind you in the palms-forward variation. These variations can be effective if the seated variations are not working well or are uncomfortable.

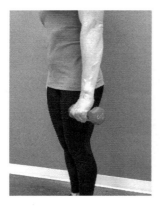 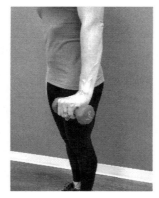 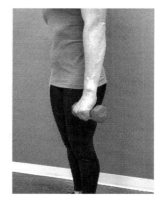

Pronation/Supination

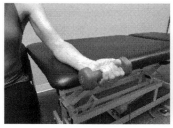 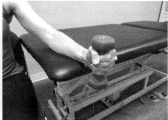 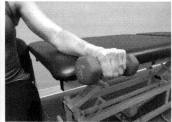 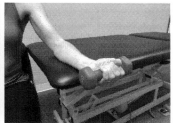

Sit in a chair and face parallel to a table with a dumbbell or, alternatively, the head of a hammer in your hand. Bend the elbow of your affected arm to a 90-degree angle and rest your forearm so your wrist is just barely off the edge of the table. Start with your palm face up and your wrist in line with your forearm so the dumbbell rotates from one side to the other (180 degrees) using the appropriate eccentric time when lowering it. Rotate back to the starting position in a controlled manner.

Although this exercise does not directly work the extensor muscles, we have found it to be particularly effective because of the incremental loading on the tendons as the forearm rotates. Therefore, it can be used as a basic exercise to introduce load to the tendon.

A pair of gymnastics rings can be particularly helpful as you are resuming upper-body strengthening exercises like pull-ups or chin-ups.

TRICEPS

Triceps Pressdowns

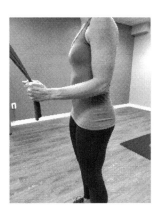 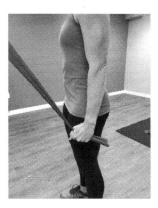 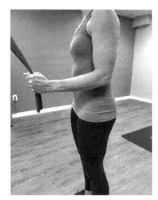

This exercise requires a band or pulley system from a gym to perform. The band or pulley must have a line of pull overhead.

Begin by grabbing the band or pulley and walk forward until it is almost vertical. Keep your arm by your side and extend your elbow until it is straight. Then, slowly allow your arm to bend again using the appropriate eccentric time.

Skullcrushers

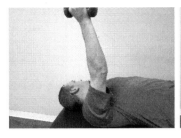 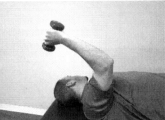 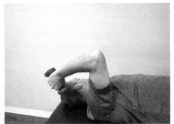 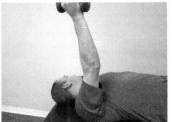

Lie on your back on a sturdy bench. Raise your arm to a 90-degree angle with your body. Then, slowly allow gravity to bend your elbow for the appropriate eccentric time. Your hand will move toward your body—hence the term "skullcrusher." Next, straighten your arm in a controlled manner to the starting position to complete the repetition.

Overhead Triceps Extension

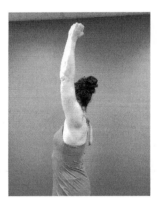 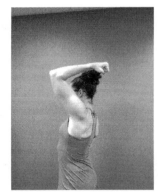 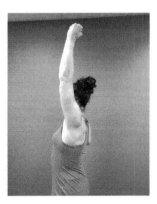

Stand up straight with your affected arm fully overhead. Slowly allow gravity to bend your arm backward, keeping your forearm in line with your head, for the appropriate eccentric time. Conclude by straightening your arm in a controlled manner to the starting position

BICEPS

Proximal

Overhead Straight-arm Lower and Raise

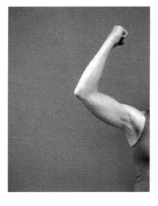 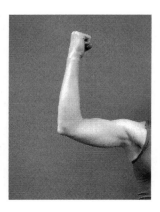 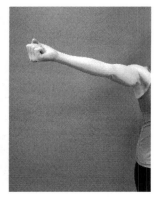

Begin in a standing position with your arm raised to an angle of roughly 120 to 150 degrees in the scaption plane (45-degrees to the side of the front raise and 45-degrees in front of the side raise) with your elbow bent at a 90-degree angle. Slowly lower your shoulder down to 90 degrees and then slowly extend your elbow until your arm is straight. Next, slowly lower your arm (against gravity) until it reaches your side. The appropriate eccentric time can be emphasized in any or multiple of the 3 phases, depending on how the proximal biceps tendon responds best.

Proximal biceps tendinopathy usually benefits from the addition of rotator cuff exercises to the rehabilitation program. In our experience, this tends to be helpful because the proximal biceps tendon connects to the superior labrum, providing some level of stability for the shoulder. Strengthening the rotator cuff muscles will increase stability for the shoulder, which will likely help to reduce the load sustained by the proximal biceps tendon.

Distal

Supinated Biceps Curls

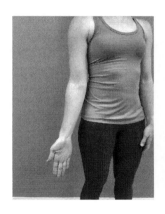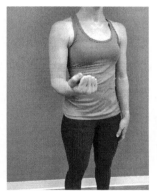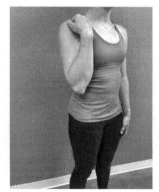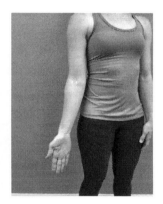

Begin in a standing position with your palm facing forward. Curl your hand upward (against gravity) until it is close to your shoulder and reaches the limit of your range of motion or until there is discomfort. Slowly lower your hand back to the starting position using the appropriate eccentric time.

Hammer Biceps Curls

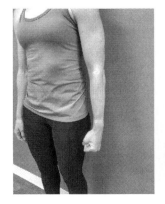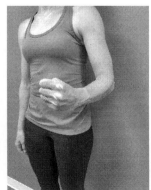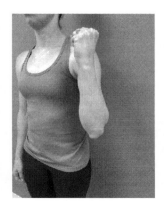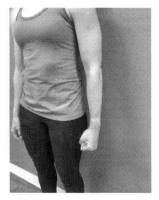

Begin in a standing position with your arm by your side and your palm facing toward your body. Curl your hand upward (against gravity) until it is close to your shoulder and reaches the limit of your range of motion or until there is discomfort. Slowly lower your hand back to the starting position using the appropriate eccentric time.

Pronated Biceps Curls

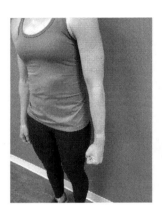 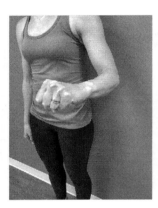 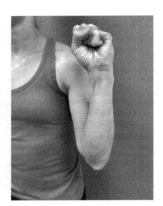

Begin in a standing position with your palm backward. Curl your hand upward (against gravity) until it is close to your shoulder and reaches the limit of your range of motion or until there is discomfort. Slowly lower your hand back to the starting position using the appropriate eccentric time.

Other variations of curls, such as decline bench curls or preacher curls, can also be used as needed to load the biceps tendon through different ranges of motion. Apply the appropriate exercise variation for your specific needs.

Supination/Pronation

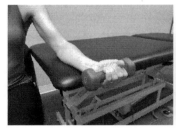 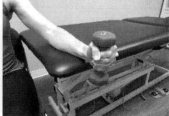 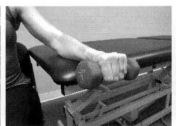 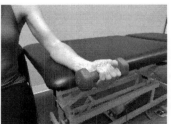

Sit in a chair and face parallel to a table with a dumbbell or, alternatively, the head of a hammer in your hand. Bend the elbow of your affected arm to a 90-degree angle and rest your forearm so your wrist is just barely off the edge of the table. Start with your palm face up and your wrist in line with your forearm so the dumbbell rotates from one side to the other (180 degrees) using the appropriate eccentric time when lowering it. Rotate back to the starting position in a controlled manner.

One of the other functions of the biceps is supination, along with the main function of elbow flexion, so this can be very useful if the variations of curls are not hitting the affected area well.

All three variations of biceps curls are shown here is because there are times when the supinated or hammer curl can aggravate distal biceps tendinopathy, even at lower intensities. To counteract this, we have found it helpful to start with pronated biceps curls and slowly transition to hammer curls. As the biceps start to decrease in pain and improve in function, you can transition from hammer curls to supinated curls. Additionally, the supination/pronation provides an eccentric distal biceps rehabilitation, as one of the functions of the biceps is to supinate the forearm. This can be used in conjunction with biceps curls or as a basic starting exercise if the biceps tendinopathy is particularly bad.

Additionally, standing biceps curls may not hit the particular area(s) effectively if the tendinopathy is aggravated in a particular range of motion, such as when the elbow is almost fully straight or bent. You may have to modify the exercises in order to hit those specific ranges, such as with preacher curls or incline bench curls, respectively, in order to place the proper rehabilitation stress on the tendon.

A pair of gymnastics rings can be particularly helpful as you are resuming upper-body strengthening exercises like pull-ups or chin-ups. This is because the rings allow for free rotation, enabling your wrists, elbows, and shoulders to avoid getting stuck in a particular movement pattern that can aggravate upper-body tendinopathies like golfer's elbow, tennis elbow, biceps, and rotator cuff tendinopathies.

ACHILLES

The two main areas of Achilles tendinopathy are insertional and mid-portion. Insertional tends to be the more problematic one to deal with because the compression of the tendon around the Achilles bursa can make the area very reactive. For this reason, mid-portion tends to lend toward better results, so clinicians need to take care to ensure insertional cases do not flare up.

Insertional Achilles

Flat Ground Calf Raises

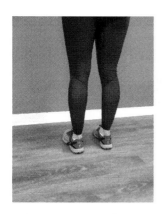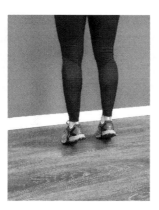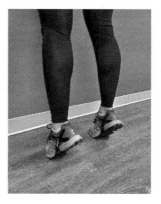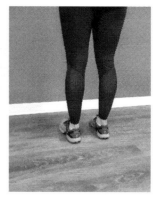

Begin in a standing position with your feet flat on the ground. Move to a wall or other sturdy implement like a table for balance (if needed). Slowly raise your heels off the ground, as high as you can, until you reach the end of your range of motion. Slowly lower your heels back to the starting position using the appropriate eccentric time.

This exercise may need to be performed with both legs at first, as those with moderate or severe tendinopathy can experience too much aggravation if they begin with just one leg. As you get stronger, you can slowly modify it to two legs with increased repetitions or weights before transitioning to one leg. Sometimes if the concentric (raising the heel off the ground) is too aggravating, you can use the non-injured side to raise up and then assist with the eccentric motion lowering to the ground slowly. Eventually, it can be progressed to a single leg.

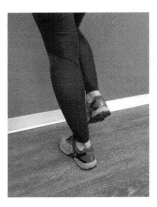 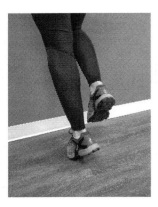 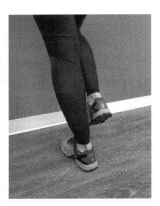

Calf Raise Machine

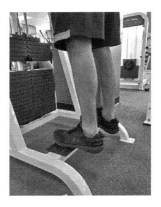 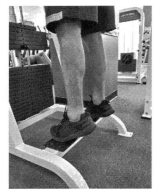 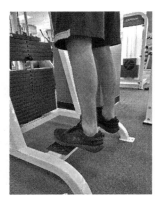

This exercise can be performed in a seated or standing position. Begin by loading the appropriate weight (if any) into the machine. Do not allow your heel to dip below the front of your foot. Slowly raise your heel off the ground, as high as you can, until you reach the end of your range of motion or experience discomfort. Slowly lower your heels back to the starting position using the appropriate eccentric time.

Mid-portion Achilles

Box/Step Calf Raises or Incline Board Calf Raises

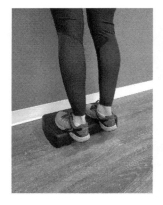 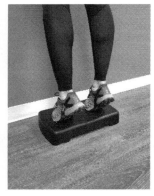 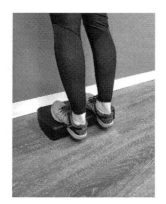 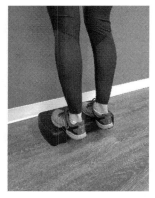

Begin by standing on a sturdy box or step. Alternatively, if you have a tilted board, stand with your toes on the uphill portion of the board and your heel on the downhill portion of the board. (If you need help balancing, move closer to a wall or other sturdy implement like a table.) Slowly raise your heels off the ground, as high as you can, until you reach the end of your range of motion. Slowly lower your heel back to the starting position using the appropriate eccentric time.

You may need to perform this exercise with both legs at first, as moderate to severe tendinopathy can be too aggravating if you only use one leg. As you get stronger, you can slowly modify the exercise with increased repetitions or weights. You may want to do this first before progressing to one leg. Sometimes, if the concentric motion (raising your heel off the ground) is too aggravating, you can use your non-injured side to raise your leg up and then assist with the eccentric motion (slowly lowering to the ground).

Here is what the single leg variation looks like:

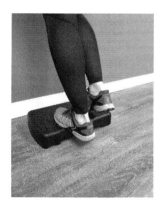 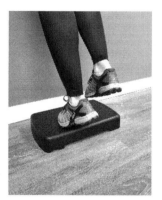 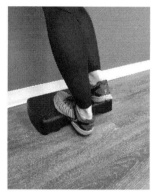 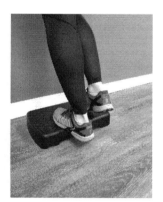

Calf Raise Machine

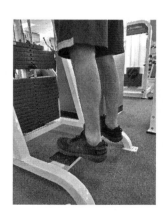 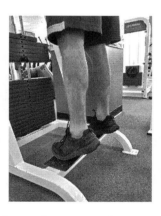 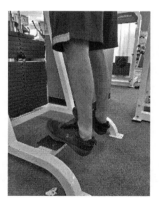 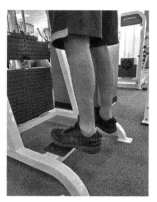

This exercise can be performed in a seated or standing position. Begin by loading the appropriate weight (if any) into the machine. Then, sit or stand at the calf raise machine and allow your heel to dip below the height of the front of the foot. Go until you reach the end of your range of motion or experience discomfort. Slowly lower your heels back to the starting position using the appropriate eccentric time.

POSTERIOR TIBIALIS

Since the posterior tibialis action is plantar flexion and inversion of the ankle, those are the specific movements that must be targeted in rehabilitation.

Calf Raises

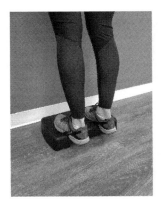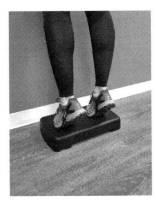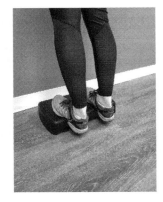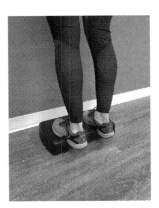

Stand with your feet flat on the ground. (If you need help balancing, move closer to a wall or other sturdy implement like a table.) Slowly raise your heels off the ground, as high as you can, until you reach the end of your range of motion. Slowly lower your heels back to the starting position using the appropriate eccentric time.

You may need to perform this exercise with both legs at first, as moderate to severe tendinopathy can be too aggravating if you only use one leg. As you get stronger, you can slowly modify the exercise with increased repetitions or weights. You may want to do this first before progressing to one leg. Sometimes, if the concentric motion (raising your heel off the ground) is too aggravating, you can use your non-injured side to raise your leg up and then assist with the eccentric motion (slowly lowering to the ground).

Here is what the single leg variation looks like:

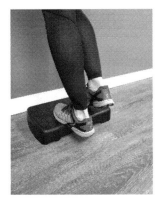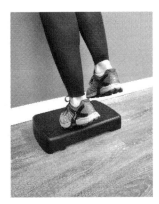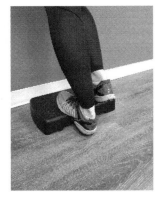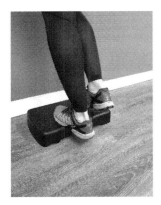

Thera-Band Ankle Inversion Eccentrics

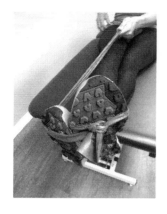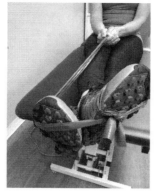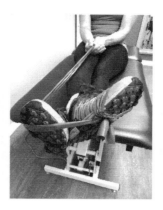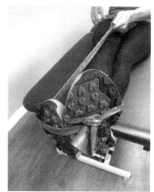

A band can be used to work inversion of the ankle. Begin by looping a band around the foot of the affected leg. Your unaffected leg should be extended straight in front of you. Place your affected leg over your unaffected leg so they are crossed and the affected leg is on top. The band should be looped around the foot of the affected leg and the toe of the unaffected leg. Rotate your foot inward toward that side's big toe. After you reach the limit of your range of motion, slowly allow the band to pull your affected foot back to the starting position using the appropriate eccentric time.

PATELLAR

Decline Board Squats

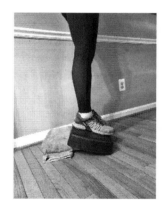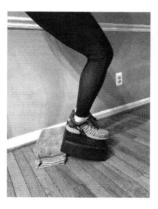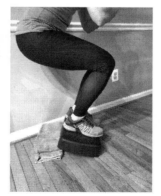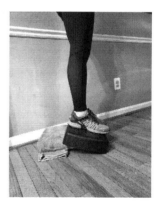

Squats on a Modified Decline Board

Begin by standing on a board with your toes on the downhill portion of the board and your heels on the uphill portion. (If you need help balancing, move closer to a wall or other sturdy implement like a table.) Slowly descend into a squat position, with your legs parallel to the ground, for the appropriate eccentric time. If you cannot reach the point where your legs are parallel to the ground, go as far as you are able. Keep your weight balanced throughout your feet and do not let your toes or heels come off the ground. It is fine for your knees to extend in front of the toes during this exercise. Ascend from the bottom of the squat position in a slow and controlled manner.

If the decline board squat is too difficult or you do not have a decline board, you can begin this exercise on a level floor. In this instance, aim to keep your knees in line with your toes and do not allow them to extend significantly beyond your toes as you squat, as this will decrease the amount of stress placed on your knees.

You can eventually progress to single-leg squats or decline board single leg squats.

Knee Extension Eccentrics

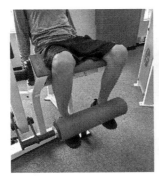 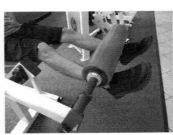 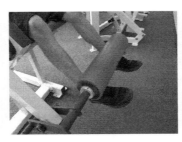 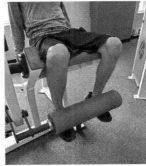

Using a knee extension machine, load the appropriate weight for your affected leg. Begin the exercise by extending your knee in a controlled fashion. (You may need to use your unaffected leg to assist. After your knee is straight, disengage your unaffected leg.) Next, slowly allow your affected leg to bend back to the starting position using the appropriate eccentric time.

Stair Step-downs

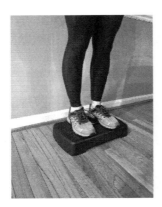 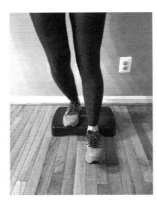 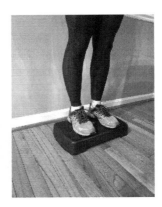

Your affected leg will be on the board, controlling the step-down.

Begin by standing on a staircase. Slowly step down to the next stair using your unaffected leg while your affected leg controls the movement. Use the appropriate eccentric time and return to your starting position. (If you need help balancing, use the railing or wall.) Next, turn around and step back up to the previous stair.

Sometimes, stepping back up with your affected leg can be aggravating, which is why we recommend turning around before stepping back up. If that is too tedious for you, you can usually start at the top of the staircase in order to get multiple repetitions of the exercise in a row without having to turn around and step back up. Another alternative is to use the railing to push off hard with your unaffected leg to step back up if this movement is bothering your affected leg.

HAMSTRINGS

Proximal Hamstring

Eccentric Hip Bridges

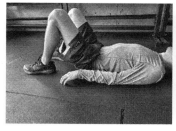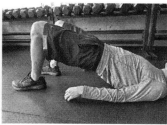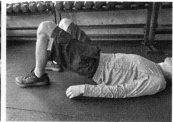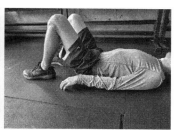

Begin by lying on your back. Bend your legs to a 90-degree angle while keeping your feet on the floor. Your butt should lift off the ground and form a straight line from your knees, through your butt, to your shoulders. Complete the movement by slowly lowering your butt to the starting position using the appropriate eccentric time.

You can add weight to the exercise by placing a dumbbell, weight plate, or barbell on your hip. Alternatively, you can progress to a single leg hip bridge as you are able.

Treadmill Backward Walking

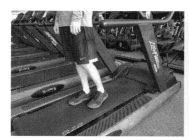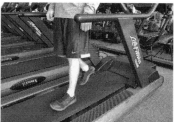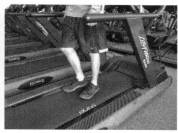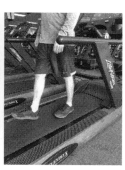

Practice walking backward on the ground first until get the hang of it. Then, start the treadmill at a very slow speed and use the handlebars to safely begin walking backward on it. Walk for a set amount of time (a few minutes) to start. Rest and repeat for additional sets. Since this is not a traditional "repetition" exercise, you must track your progress by speed and time.

The reason this exercise only works on a treadmill as opposed to the ground is because the treadmill is moving, which forces the eccentric lengthening of the hamstring as the treadmill moves your foot away from your body. On the ground, the mechanics of walking backward are not the same, as you must lean back and push off with your foot which does not eccentrically work your hamstring.

Romanian Deadlift

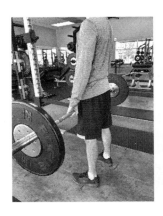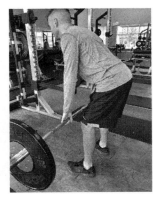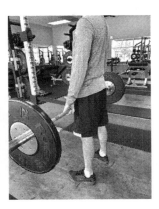

Begin in a standing position with an overhand grip on dumbbells or a barbell. Slowly lower toward the ground, keeping your back straight and chest up while bending your knees, for the appropriate eccentric time. Once the dumbbells or barbell reach the height of the knees, ascend in a controlled manner to the starting position.

If eccentric hip bridges and treadmill backward walking are not working to effectively rehabilitate your proximal hamstring, Romanian deadlifts can be a good alternative. This exercise emphasizes the hamstrings in a hip hinge, which is helpful to target the proximal hamstring origin that can sometimes be difficult to rehabilitate. However, the movement can be a bit technical to perform, so make sure you are getting proper coaching before trying it out yourself if you are not aware of how to do the correct form.

This exercise can be progressed by lowering the bar to go an inch or two from touching the ground.

Distal Hamstring

Prone Leg Curl Eccentrics

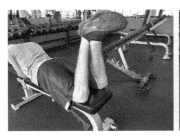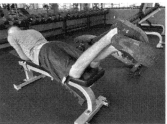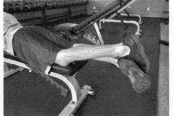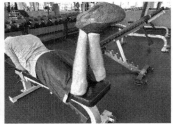

Lie on your stomach with your affected leg bent at a 90-degree angle. (If you need more resistance, add an ankle weight.) Slowly lower your leg utilizing the appropriate eccentric time. (You may need to use your unaffected leg to assist.) After your knee is straight, disengage your unaffected leg if you were using it for assistance. Slowly contract your hamstring to bring your affected leg back to the starting position.

If you do not have any ankle weights or bands, you can use your unaffected leg to provide resistance. In the images above, the affected leg is on the right while the left leg pushes into the right leg to provide additional resistance for the eccentric-concentric movement.

Machine Leg Curl Eccentrics

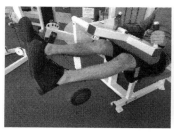 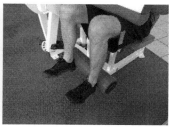 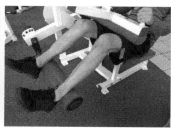 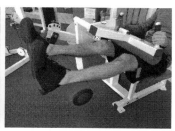

Using a leg curl machine, load the appropriate weight for your affected leg. Begin the exercise by curling your knee in a controlled fashion. (You may need to use your unaffected leg to assist.) After your knee is bent to a 90-degree angle or greater, disengage your unaffected leg if you were using it for assistance. Slowly allow your affected leg to straighten back to the starting position while performing the appropriate eccentric time.

CHAPTER 8

OUTCOME MEASURES AND INTERVENTION CHARTS

TENDINOPATHY INTERVENTION CHARTS, BLURBS, ABBREVIATIONS, AND EXPLANATIONS

We constructed these intervention charts to help patients and clinicians determine their options regarding the effectiveness of various treatment options for tendinopathy. While reviewing the scientific literature, we found something interesting: at times, the evidence varied from one body part to another.

We categorized these intervention charts into "major" and "minor" interventions based on the paucity of the research. For the interventions where we found more research, we constructed major charts that include our general recommendations, any potential adverse effects, the most prevalent outcome measures to track rehabilitation, and any other comments. For the minor interventions with less or lacking research, we provided a simple summary based on what was available.

We gave preference to systematic reviews and meta-analyses over randomized controlled trials (RCTs), and RCTs over the rest of the studies. This is based on the evidence categorization in Chapter 1. A lot of the research is convoluted or inconsistent and many of the studies seem to have poor methodology or risk of bias, so the conclusions are weak, at best, much of the time.

Here are the major interventions we will cover:

- Eccentric Loading and Exercise Therapy
- Corticosteroid Injections (CST)
- Extracorporeal Shockwave Therapy (ECST or ESWT)
- Low-Level Laser Therapy (LLLT)
- Platelet-rich Plasma (PRP), Autologous Blood Injection (ABI), and Prolotherapy
- Therapeutic Ultrasound
- Surgery

Here are the minor interventions we will cover:

- Botulinum Toxin (Botox)
- Ergonomics
- Iontophoresis

- Manual Therapy / Massage
- Needling Techniques (Acupuncture, Dry Needling, etc.)
- Nitroglycerin/Nitric Oxide/Glyceryl Trinitrate (GTN)
- Pain Medication
- Stretching Exercises
- Supplements
- Transcutaneous Electrical Nerve Stimulation (TENS)
- Wait and See (also called Watchful Waiting)
- Calcific Tendinopathy
- Bracing

Here is a list of abbreviations we will use:

- AT—Achilles Tendinopathy
- PT—Patellar Tendinopathy
- LET—Lateral Elbow Tendinopathy
- HS—Hamstring Tendinopathy
- RCT—Rotator Cuff Tendinopathy
- Other—Other Tendinopathies

We listed the remaining tendinopathies, such as medial elbow, posterior tibialis, wrist, etc. as "other tend-inopathies" because they are not as common as the ones discussed above.

All references for each of these charts and blurbs are listed in the endnotes section at the end of this book. We initially wanted to place them next to each reference, but it quickly made the book quite messy when they were coupled with the charts themselves.

Please use discretion before referring to anything indicated in this chapter as "gospel truth." We recommend reading the studies cited in the endnotes and coming to your own conclusions.

GRADE OF EVIDENCE

As seen in Chapter 1, the levels of evidence range from I to V, based on quality, and A to F, based on the effectiveness of the intervention. The A to F scale ranged from stronger, moderate, weak, conflicting, theoretical, and expert opinion.

To make the charts as uncomplicated as possible, we went with a modified version consisting of strong, moderate, weak, and no evidence. Then, we used these levels of evidence to categorize the general effect: favorable, limited, no effect, mixed (conflicting), or negative.

- Favorable—The intervention has a positive effect on tendinopathy.
- Limited—The intervention *may* have a slight positive effect. In most cases, more studies are warranted.
- No effect—The intervention has no effect on tendinopathy.
- Mixed—The intervention has no effect in some studies and a slight positive effect in others. In most cases, more studies are warranted.
- Negative—The intervention has a negative effect on tendinopathy and, usually, makes it worse.

As we noted earlier in this section, the levels of evidence for each of these were mostly drawn from level I (systematic reviews, high-quality diagnostic, prospective or randomized controlled trials) and level II (lower-quality studies with weaker criteria or improper randomization) studies with some level III, IV, and V studies if there was very little on the particular intervention. Since Achilles and Patellar are the most commonly studied tendinopathy, the evidence levels tended to be stronger compared to other tendinopathies. Some, like hamstring, tended to have weak evidence since very few studies have been conducted.

MAJOR
INTERVENTIONS

Eccentrics
SUMMARY OF EFFECTIVENESS

	Favorable	Limited	No Effect	Mixed	Negative
Achilles Mid-portion	Fav	Lim	No	Mix	Neg
Pain	●				
Function	●				
Short-Term	●				
Long-Term	◐				
Achilles Insertional	Fav	Lim	No	Mix	Neg
Pain		◐			
Function		○			
Short-Term		◐			
Long-Term				○	
Patellar	Fav	Lim	No	Mix	Neg
Pain	●				
Function		●			
Short-Term	●				
Long-Term	◐				
Lateral Epicondylitis	Fav	Lim	No	Mix	Neg
Pain	◐				
Function	◐				
Short-Term	●				
Long-Term	○				

	Favorable	Limited	No Effect	Mixed	Negative
Proximal Hamstring	Fav	Lim	No	Mix	Neg
Pain	○				
Function	○				
Short-Term	○				
Long-Term	○				
Adductor	Fav	Lim	No	Mix	Neg
Pain	◐				
Function		◐			
Short-Term	◐				
Long-Term	◐				
Rotator Cuff	Fav	Lim	No	Mix	Neg
Pain		◐			
Function	◐				
Short-Term	◐				
Long-Term					

Evidence:

Strong	●
Moderate	◐
Weak	○
None	----

Recommendations

As we have discussed, *eccentric loading* (especially that which is combined with concentric loading) of an injured tendon plays an important role in its return to normal functioning ability. Eccentric loading programs are essentially the only intervention found to have a strong body of evidence for beneficial effects for tendinopathies, particularly for Achilles and patellar tendons. Much of the scientific literature we reviewed seemed to agree that an eccentric loading program should be the "gold standard" intervention for tendon issues and, in most circumstances, the first treatment attempted before others are considered. There also seems to be a greater beneficial effect for a variety of other interventions when eccentrics are added to them.

We recommend utilizing an eccentric-concentric loading program for any tendon issues diagnosed as the first option in order to promote both short-term and long-term tendon healing and return to normal functioning ability. Other interventions may assist in pain relief and other short-term benefits, but should not be chosen in place of eccentric-concentric exercises.

If you'd like to review our specific recommendations for achieving optimal performance from each tendon area, see the concentric-eccentric rehabilitation section of Chapter 4.

Adverse Effects

- Delayed onset muscle soreness (DOMS)

Most Prevalent Outcome Measures

All	VAS, MMT
Achilles	VISA-A, LEFS
Patellar	VISA-P
Shoulder	DASH
Elbow	TEFS, elbow disability

Other Comments

- Evidence suggests there is no need to fully withdraw from sports activity during eccentric exercise training. Coaches or physical therapists may need to modify the frequency, intensity, or volume of the sport-specific exercises in order to decrease the potential to aggravate or worsen the tendon during rehabilitation.
- Measurements of tendon thickness does not seem to correlate with clinical, symptomatic outcomes.
- A systematic review on Achilles eccentric protocols favors the Alfredson protocol, which includes 3x15 full-range calf raises performed three times per day at bent and straight knee positions. Other reviews may prefer HSR for patellar. The program used falls under the clinician's discretion. See Chapter 6 for further details.

Corticosteroidal Injections (CST)

SUMMARY OF EFFECTIVENESS

	Favorable	Limited	No Effect	Mixed	Negative
Achilles Mid-portion	Fav	Lim	No	Mix	Neg
Pain		●			
Function					●
Short-Term				●	
Long-Term					●
Achilles Insertional	Fav	Lim	No	Mix	Neg
Pain	○				
Function	—	—	—	—	—
Short-Term	○				
Long-Term	—	—	—	—	—
Patellar	Fav	Lim	No	Mix	Neg
Pain	●				
Function		●			
Short-Term	●				
Long-Term		○			
Lateral Epicondylitis	Fav	Lim	No	Mix	Neg
Pain	●				
Function				●	
Short-Term	●				
Long-Term					●

	Favorable	Limited	No Effect	Mixed	Negative
Rotator Cuff	Fav	Lim	No	Mix	Neg
Pain	●				
Function				●	
Short-Term	●				
Long-Term					●
Medial Epicondylitis	Fav	Lim	No	Mix	Neg
Pain			○		
Function	—	—	—	—	—
Short-Term			○		
Long-Term	—	—	—	—	—

Evidence:

Strong	●
Moderate	●
Weak	○
None	—

Recommendations

Steroid injections (also referred to as *corticosteroids*) are a concerning intervention for tendon injuries. There is substantial evidence that corticosteroids have a weakening effect on tendons over time, to the point of tendon rupture, particularly when they are used consistently over an extended period of time. At the same time, there is significant evidence that steroid injections have a favorable short-term effect on painful tendon issues with no significant beneficial long-term effect (and possible negative effects).

We still recommend seeking other short-term interventions for pain management, but if those fail and there is a significant function deficit due to pain, a corticosteroid injection treatment may be an option. One or two injections may help pain tolerance while implementing other interventions to address tendon healing without risking major adverse effects. Any more than that seems to result in minor to major adverse long-term effects.

Adverse Effects

- Higher risk of tendon weakness and/or rupture related to long-term use
- Joint infection
- Nerve damage
- Bone deficiency

Most Prevalent Outcome Measures

All	VAS
Achilles	VISA-A, Pain pressure threshold, response to tx, ultrasound tendon diameter
Patellar	Pain pressure threshold, response to tx
Elbow	DASH, patient perceived change, NRS pain/function, PRFEQ pain/function
Shoulder	DASH, Shoulder disability questionnaire, Oxford shoulder score

Other Comments

- Many studies suggest steroidal injections are just as effective at relieving pain as NSAIDs.
- One systematic review states steroidal injections may have a longer lasting benefit for rotator cuff tendonitis.
- Ultrasound guided injections may be more accurate.

Extracorporeal Shockwave Therapy
SUMMARY OF EFFECTIVENESS

	Favorable	Limited	No Effect	Mixed	Negative
Achilles Mid-portion	Fav	Lim	No	Mix	Neg
Pain		●			
Function		●			
Short-Term		●			
Long-Term		●			
Achilles Insertional	Fav	Lim	No	Mix	Neg
Pain	●				
Function		●			
Short-Term	●				
Long-Term		●			
Patellar	Fav	Lim	No	Mix	Neg
Pain		●			
Function				●	
Short-Term		●			
Long-Term				●	

	Favorable	Limited	No Effect	Mixed	Negative
Lateral Epicondylitis	Fav	Lim	No	Mix	Neg
Pain	●				
Function		●			
Short-Term	●				
Long-Term		●			
Rotator Cuff	Fav	Lim	No	Mix	Neg
Pain	●				
Function		●			
Short-Term	●				
Long-Term	●				
Proximal Hamstring	Fav	Lim	No	Mix	Neg
Pain		○			
Function		○			
Short-Term		○			
Long-Term					

Evidence:

Strong	●
Moderate	●
Weak	○
None	---

Recommendations

Extracorporeal shockwave therapy shows a favorable, though limited, body of evidence regarding tendon issues. We found some intriguing evidence as to its positive effect for sites and the change for continued, long-term positive effects. ESWT also has a fairly extensive research base that exceeds many of the other interventions studied. However, a more recent review discovered there is a high risk of bias in much of the earlier research concerning ESWT's effectiveness.

Because of this, we recommend using this method with caution, and only after more proven measures—such as eccentric loading—have been attempted. However, we would recommend this over other, riskier methods like surgical intervention.

Adverse Effects

- Reddening of the skin
- Pain
- Small hematomas

Most Prevalent Outcome Measures

All	VAS
Achilles	VISA-A, Likert, NRS, pain threshold, AOFAS, FIL, AHS
Patellar	VISA-P, Likert, vertical jump test, AOFAS, FIL
Elbow	DASH, UEFS, Roles and Maudsley scale
Shoulder	subjective patient satisfaction, Constant and Murley scale (CMS), UCLA scale

Other Comments

- Many studies recommend adding an eccentric loading program to laser ESWT due to potential accelerated benefits.
- There seems to be a consensus that ESWT has a higher potential positive effect on calcific tendon sites like insertional Achilles and rotator cuff regions.
- ESWT is, in many cases, the most expensive option of all the major treatment interventions.

Low-Level Laser Therapy (LLLT)

SUMMARY OF EFFECTIVENESS

Achilles Mid-portion	Favorable	Limited	No Effect	Mixed	Negative
Pain				●	
Function				○	
Short-Term				●	
Long-Term				○	

Achilles Insertional	Fav	Lim	No	Mix	Neg
Pain		○			
Function		—			
Short-Term		○			
Long-Term		○			

Lateral Epicondylitis	Fav	Lim	No	Mix	Neg
Pain		●			
Function				○	
Short-Term		●			
Long-Term			○		

Rotator Cuff	Fav	Lim	No	Mix	Neg
Pain		?		○	
Function				○	
Short-Term		?		○	
Long-Term				○	

Adductor	Fav	Lim	No	Mix	Neg
Pain			○		
Function			○		
Short-Term			○		
Long-Term			○		

Evidence:

Strong	●
Moderate	●
Weak	○
None	—

Recommendations

The evidence for *low-level laser therapy* is quite diverse due to the large number of variables involved in treatment techniques. Differences can be found regarding wavelength applied, number of treatment sessions, time between treatments, and application techniques. Because of this, many conflicting conclusions are drawn, and the strength of evidence is generally weak. It seems there is weak to moderate evidence for short-term pain relief benefits for insertional Achilles and elbow tendinopathies (over other areas), but the benefits for function were less convincing.

There are virtually no adverse effects and it is relatively cost-effective, which is why it is seems to be an increasingly marketable option; however, we'd caution against using this as a long-term solution since tendon healing properties are lacking. We recommend it as a potential option for short-term pain relief in conjunction with eccentric-concentric rehabilitation exercises, particularly if other pain-relieving options have failed.

Adverse Effects

- Eye injury (if you look directly into the light beam)

Most Prevalent Outcome Measures

All	VAS
Achilles	VISA-A
Elbow	PRTEE, pain-pressure threshold, pain free grip strength
Shoulder	Constant and Murley score (CMS)

Other Comments

- Many studies recommend adding an eccentric loading program to laser therapy due to potential accelerated benefits.
- Multiple studies suggest the best wavelength range is between 810 and 904nm, with 904nm being the most preferred.

Platelet-rich Plasma (PRP), Autologous blood injection (ABI), and Prolotherapy

SUMMARY OF EFFECTIVENESS

	Favorable	Limited	No Effect	Mixed	Negative

Achilles Mid-portion	Fav	Lim	No	Mix	Neg
Pain		?		●	
Function			●		
Short-Term		?		●	
Long-Term				○	

Achilles Insertional	Fav	Lim	No	Mix	Neg
Pain				○	
Function					
Short-Term				○	
Long-Term		—	—	—	

Patellar	Fav	Lim	No	Mix	Neg
Pain		●			
Function		●			
Short-Term		●			
Long-Term		●			

Lateral Epicondylitis	Fav	Lim	No	Mix	Neg
Pain		?		●	
Function			●		
Short-Term				●	
Long-Term		?		●	

Proximal Hamstring	Fav	Lim	No	Mix	Neg
Pain		○			
Function		○			
Short-Term		○			
Long-Term		—	—	—	

Rotator Cuff	Fav	Lim	No	Mix	Neg
Pain				●	
Function				○	
Short-Term				●	
Long-Term				●	

Evidence:

Strong	● (black)
Moderate	● (gray)
Weak	○
None	—

Recommendations

Platelet-rich plasma, autologous blood injections, and *prolotherapy* are similar enough interventions in mechanism that we thought it appropriate to combine their results in the context of tendon injury. Out of the major interventions we reviewed for the charts, it is difficult to make general recommendations for these interventions because increased research has yielded conflicting results. Some research suggests these treatment methods are potentially beneficial. However, the overall effect seems to be limited. Still others say these methods are of no benefit whatsoever.

Our recommendation is that these injectable therapies should not be the first option for tendon treatment, but could be considered for Achilles, patellar, and elbow areas if more conservative options are first exhausted. Research is limited as to how these treatments could benefit other areas so we are unable to make further recommendations. If this intervention is chosen, it should be paired with additional treatments, such as an eccentric-concentric loading program.

Adverse Effects

- Skin itchiness
- Transient pain post-needling

Most Prevalent Outcome Measures

All	VAS, patient satisfaction scales
Achilles	VISA-A
Elbow	PRTEE, pain-pressure threshold
Shoulder	DASH

Other Comments

- Some evidence suggests platelet injections may be more beneficial to assist with the healing of ruptured tendons over tendinopathies.
- A few studies found PRP injections are more effective for females than males. However, an explanation was not given.

Therapeutic Ultrasound
SUMMARY OF EFFECTIVENESS

Achilles Mid-portion	Fav	Lim	No	Mix	Neg
Pain			○		
Function			○		
Short-Term			○		
Long-Term	—	—	—	—	—
Patellar	Fav	Lim	No	Mix	Neg
Pain			●		
Function			○		
Short-Term			●		
Long-Term	—	—	—	—	—
Lateral Epicondylitis	Fav	Lim	No	Mix	Neg
Pain				●	
Function			●		
Short-Term				●	
Long-Term			●		

Medial Epicondylitis	Fav	Lim	No	Mix	Neg
Pain			○		
Function			○		
Short-Term			○		
Long-Term			○		
Rotator Cuff	Fav	Lim	No	Mix	Neg
Pain				●	
Function			●		
Short-Term			●		
Long-Term			●		

Evidence:	
Strong	●
Moderate	●
Weak	○
None	—

Recommendations

Therapeutic ultrasound (as opposed to ultrasound guidance techniques used for diagnostic or intervention purposes) is a household name and staple in the pain relief world and has been since the 1950s. Unfortunately, there is not a wealth of research evidence on its general effectiveness and the evidence that does exist suggests that it's not very effective in relation to tendinopathies. Both Achilles and patellar tendon issues seem to not respond at all to ultrasound, whereas elbow and shoulder tendon response is conflicting: some studies reveal a small, short-term benefit while other studies show it to be of no effect. Adverse effects are mild and uncommon, which is likely one of the reasons it is so prevalent.

We do not recommend therapeutic ultrasound at all for tendon issues. We believe its effectiveness to be no more than a placebo effect, and a cost-benefit analysis of both the medical provider's time and the patient's time and money is poor. The only instance where we would recommend it would be prior to considering surgery once all other upper-body tendinopathy treatment options have been exhausted.

Adverse Effects

- Can burn the skin if left in one area for too long

Most Prevalent Outcome Measures

All	VAS
Achilles	VISA-A
Patellar	VISA-P
Elbow	pain free grip strength
Shoulder	DASH

Other Comments

- One systematic review not only concluded the benefits of therapeutic ultrasound are no better than a placebo effect, but it also fails to enhance the effectiveness of exercise.
- One study suggested a potentially positive effect for calcific rotator cuff tendinopathy specifically.
- One study claimed potential benefits for cryoultrasound when used to treat insertional Achilles tendinopathy.

Surgery
SUMMARY OF EFFECTIVENESS

Achilles Mid-portion	Fav	Lim	No	Mix	Neg
Pain		●		●	
Function		●			●
Short-Term		●			
Long-Term				●	

Achilles Insertional	Fav	Lim	No	Mix	Neg
Pain		●			
Function		●			●
Short-Term		●			
Long-Term		●			

Patellar	Fav	Lim	No	Mix	Neg
Pain		●		●	
Function		●		●	
Short-Term		●			
Long-Term		●			

Lateral Epicondylitis	Fav	Lim	No	Mix	Neg
Pain		○			○
Function		○			○
Short-Term		○			
Long-Term		○			

Rotator Cuff	Fav	Lim	No	Mix	Neg
Pain	●				
Function		●			●
Short-Term	●				
Long-Term		●			

Proximal Hamstring	Fav	Lim	No	Mix	Neg
Pain		○			
Function		○			○
Short-Term		○			
Long-Term		○			

Evidence:

Strong	●
Moderate	●
Weak	○
None	—

Recommendations

Surgery should be an absolute last resort for all tendon areas. There is an inherent risk with choosing any type of surgery as there is a gaurantee of some sort of tissue damage due to the invasiveness of it. Tendon surgery is no different. The majority of surgeries turn out to be successful cases, but there will be a percentage of patients who won't have any change of symptoms post-surgery or will have significant side effects. Because these complications can often be unavoidable, we conclude that the reward does not outweigh the risk. Hence why we deem this a "last resort." Many studies conclude that surgery outcomes are no better than conservative interventions, particularly when compared to guided exercise. Additionally, it remains unclear to us and an overwhelming body of research how the excision of degenerative tissue areas affects vascularity for healing and provides resolution of pain. It is our opinion that patience, commitment, and rest are important factors in allowing a tendon to heal or become asymptomatic. If a concerted effort of time and commitment has been made, all other available measures have been exhausted, and pain persists to a level where daily functioning is affected, only then should tendon surgery be considered.

Adverse Effects

- Deep vein thrombosis (DVT)
- Nerve and muscle damage
- Wound breakdown
- Re-operation
- Frozen shoulder
- Potential to be unable to return to level of sports activity before surgery

Most Prevalent Outcome Measures

All	VAS, patient satisfaction scales
Lower extremity	VISA-A, VISA-P, LEFS
Upper extremity	DASH

Other Comments

- Surgery of the Achilles tendon is the most researched and performed type of tendon surgery. The current success rate is approximately 75 percent.

- Surgery may be less beneficial overall for non-athletes, possibly because the non-degenerative portion of the tendon has already been exercise-conditioned in athletes to bear any extra loading that the excised portion used to handle.

- There is no consensus for the best surgical techniques for many tendon areas, particularly insertional Achilles issues.

- In one systematic review, surgery was superior to no treatment or placebo, but it had similar effects to sham or "fake" surgery. This review also revealed that healthcare professionals who treat tendinopathy encouraged patients to first try loading exercise treatment for a minimum of one year before they seriously entertain the option of surgery.

MINOR
INTERVENTIONS

Botox (Botulinim Toxin)

The intended use of *botulinum toxin*, more commonly called *botox*, for medical issues involves the injection of a neurotoxin protein that comes from the bacterium clostridium botulinum. The neurotoxin shuts down the release of acetylcholine, which produces local muscle paralysis. It is theorized that the paralysis of the muscles may lead to a reduction in continuous muscle tension on tendons with poor load tolerance which may also increase pain relief.

Pros	Cons
• relatively few and generally mild side effects if administered correctly • quick and convenient procedure	• expensive procedure • possible muscle weakness at the injection site for an extended period of time • potential allergen • needles can be painful • can cause long-term complications if administered incorrectly.

Tendon-specific Research

AT   Moderate evidence that botox is not significantly better at improving pain and function than placebo.

LET   Moderate evidence that botox provides short-term pain relief for LET when compared to placebo, but can also cause extensor weakness of the wrist and fingers. Limited evidence that botox is not as effective as corticosteroids for pain relief in the short-term.

RCT   Limited evidence that botox provides short-term pain relief for RTC tendinopathy, though not as effective as CST injections. No significant long-term effectiveness for pain or function.

Items to note

Botox procedures are also commonly used for cosmetic purposes and it is important to know these instances are different from medical and pain relief use. Be aware of the services offered when seeking professional care.

Final recommendation

Botox can be an option for upper-extremity tendon issues if other approaches are proven to be ineffective. Evidence suggests there are short-term pain-relieving properties for the elbow and shoulder areas but not for the Achilles tendon. Due to the possibility of extended muscle weakness, caution should be taken if athletic or professional function is a high priority.

Ergonomics

Ergonomics refers to the study of the physical interaction between workers and their environment in hopes of improving health conditions. This is often affiliated with discussions on how the body is affected by prolonged posture, workstation setup, and computer/screen use.

Pros	Cons
• could be covered by company expenses • could have other health benefits if it promotes reduced sitting time	• can be difficult or inconvenient to adapt to new postures and positions

Tendon-specific Research

LET	Lack of high quality evidence to make an informed opinion.
RCT	Weak evidence to suggest overuse and increased vibration at work can cause shoulder tendonitis.
Other	Thumb/DeQuervian's - Limited evidence to suggest there is a causal relationship between ergonomics and DeQuervian's tenosynovitis.

Items to Note

There is an overall lack of high-quality systematic reviews linking poor ergonomics and tendon-specific issues. Much of the research we found discusses generalized or chronic issues like back, shoulder, and neck pain.

Final recommendation

It is wise to seek consultation on ergonomic changes in the workplace for general health considerations. However, we cannot make an informed recommendation on specific, tendon-related issues due to a lack of high-quality research. Much of the research guiding the medical community for this intervention is dated and a need for updated, high-quality studies is evident.

Iontophoresis

Iontophoresis is a form of medication that uses mild electrical current to drive charged molecules through the skin and into underlying tissues.

Pros	Cons
• can be self administered after learning from a health professional • very specific localization of treatment • technically non-invasive	• can result in skin alterations or reactions such as rashes, burns, and itchiness

Tendon-specific Research

AT Weak evidence iontophoresis had a favorable effect with pain and function at 6 months for Achilles tendinosis.

LET Limited evidence suggests effective when compared to placebo for pain relief in the very short term, but at 1 month there was found to be no difference. No significant effect for function was found.

RCT Weak evidence iontophoresis with acetic acid had no significant effect on calcific rotator cuff tendinopathy.

Items to note

Commonly used medications are dexamathasone, sodium diclofenac, and sodium salicylate. One study suggests sodium diclofenac may be more effective than sodium salicylate.

Final recommendation

There seems to be moderate evidence that it is useful for acute tendon pain (See the Neeter study for protocol). However, the evidence is weak to limited in cases of chronic tendon pain.

Although it is relatively easy to use and adverse effects are generally mild, we only recommend using iontophoresis for acute Achilles tendon pain, at clinician discretion, if other treatments have failed. The applicability for acute Achilles pain to other tendinopathies has not been studied but is recommended at clinician's discretion as well.

Manual Therapy / Massage

Manual therapy is a broad term for the application of physical touch by another person in order to provide pain relief and increase muscle pliability and joint mobility. This is usually performed by a licensed health professional, such as a physical, occupational, or massage therapist. *Massage* is a type of manual therapy that is most often sought out for pain and tension relief and most commonly performed on muscle tissue. One form of massage often used for tendinopathy is deep transverse friction massage, which is massage that is performed on the tendon itself, but not the muscle. The research related to tendinopathy often combines manual therapy and massage, so we will discuss them as a group.

Pros	Cons
• relatively cost-effective and convenient • most (but not all) techniques can promote relaxation • minimal risk and side effects (like temporary soreness) when proper techniques are used	• certain techniques can be somewhat painful or uncomfortable if the body's sensitivity is heightened or the force applied is too great • may need to be applied over a long period of time depending on the degree and state of injury

Tendon-specific Research

AT   Limited evidence supporting eccentric exercise as being more beneficial than deep friction massage for Achilles tendinosis alone.

LET/ MET   Moderate to strong evidence suggests manual therapy (including mobilization and manipulation) added to concentric/eccentric exercise training has a favorable effect on pain and function for both lateral and medial elbow tendinopathy. Deep transverse friction massage, however, does not seem to have a beneficial effect compared to other standard therapies for LET pain, function, and grip strength. It may have some added benefit when combined with other interventions.

RCT   There is conflicting evidence to suggest manual therapy performed on RCT can improve symptoms. If there is an effect, it would likely be for pain relief only and it is unclear if there is a significant benefit for function.

OTHER   Moderate evidence states deep transverse friction massage does not have a significant benefit compared to standard therapy exercises for iliotibial band friction syndrome at the lateral knee.

Items to Note

Manual therapy and massage treatments have an inherently high degree of variability due to skill and technique differences from one practitioner to another. There are too many techniques to count, making it quite difficult for researchers to compare one to another effectively.

Final recommendation

Manual therapy is a broad, complicated category that encompasses many different techniques, some of which have been more well-studied than others.

- Manual therapy seems to help when used in conjunction with other interventions, such as eccentric exercise protocols. The strongest evidence of this at a particular tendon area is at the elbow, where standard manual techniques and joint manipulation seem to be helpful.
- Massage of muscle tissue seems to be helpful for symptom reduction, but not necessarily for tendon healing, which can be helpful for reactive tendons.
- Deep cross friction massage was once a popular technique for tendon issues, but research has shown that it is not significantly more beneficial than standard manual and exercise interventions. We do not recommend using this intervention.
- There is some promise in the area of ASTYM therapy—but not in instrument assisted soft tissue mobilization (IASTM)—though there is not yet enough evidence for us to decide on its effectiveness, as there is only one systematic review with many of the studies being case reports. However, it is worth a try if more conservative treatment options have failed because the promising results show it is seemingly effective when paired with eccentric-concentric interventions.

Overall, we recommend adding standard manual therapy and muscle tissue massage. Though the intervention may not actually improve the load tolerance of the tendon (which is why it should be paired with eccentric-concentric interventions), the potential reduction in symptoms, promotion of muscle relaxation, and increased flexibility during exercise can help to keep patients motivated to improve and complete their rehabilitation programs. There is not much risk involved, and there is potential for a beneficial response.

Needling Techniques (Acupuncture, dry needling, etc.)

There are two interventions that utilize monofilament needles inserted under the skin in an attempt to produce positive tendon changes. *Acupuncture* is a traditional technique based on Chinese philosophical medicine that involves supposed body energy focused in points throughout the body known as "qi." Acupuncture is considered an "alternative medicine" but has a more extensive body of research compared to other needle-based treatment. The second most common needle technique is *trigger-point dry needling* (TDN), which is based in musculoskeletal theory and attempts to break up taut bands of muscle that can cause nervous system stimulation and pain. TDN is relatively new in practice and thus has a small body of research. Neither intervention claims to inject any substances; it is the needle itself that provides the benefit.

Pros	Cons
• fairly quick and convenient procedure, potentially covered by private health insurance • provides a "novel stimulus" that can have a positive effect on the nervous system • can have a relaxing or "releasing" effect	• costly if not covered by insurance • some needling techniques can have significant adverse effects if performed incorrectly • potentially painful procedure (particularly with TDN)

Tendon-specific Research

AT   Moderate evidence that acupuncture, combined with eccentric exercise, is effective for short-term pain and function of Achilles tendinopathy. Limited evidence that acupuncture can be superior to eccentric exercises for AT for less but not more than sixteen weeks. Limited evidence that eccentrics plus TDN only has a positive effect on short-term pain and function.

PT   Weak evidence to support TDN for a long-term positive effect on patellar pain.

LET   Moderate evidence that acupuncture has a positive effect over placebo and ultrasound in the short-term (two to four weeks), but not at three or twelve months for pain, function, and grip strength. Weak evidence that acupuncture has a better pain effect for LET than CST, NSAIDs and ultrasound.

RCT   Limited evidence that acupuncture has a positive short-term effect on RCT issues, not significant in the long-term for pain and function. Limited evidence that TDN only has a positive effect from baseline to six months.

Items to Note

There are different methods of both acupuncture and TDN, such as manual and electrode connection, but it is inconclusive which is the best method. Acupuncture can also be performed on a superficial or deep basis and there is limited evidence that deep is the more effective of the two.

Final recommendation

Traditional acupuncture could have short-term benefits for upper-extremity tendon issues, but only as an alternative when other treatments prove ineffective. Acupuncture and TDN could be potentially effective as an adjunct to exercise for lower-extremity tendon injuries. TDN has a more recent body of evidence that shows intriguing, positive results, but more research needs to be performed in all tendon areas.

Nitroglycerine/Nitric Oxide/Glyceryl Trinitrate (GTN)

The use of *glyceryl trinitrate* for pain has been common in multiple medical fields for decades. More recently, it has been applied to tendon injuries. It involves applying a topical patch over the most painful area of the skin that typically must be re-applied daily for a few weeks. Nitric oxide has been shown to be involved in tissue healing and collagen formation in studies involving lab rats, but the mechanism of action is still unclear.

Pros	Cons
• inexpensive, convenient and easy to apply	• headaches are a very common side effect (sometimes strong enough to cause one to cease treatment) • contact dermatitis is a less common side effect

Tendon-specific Research

AT Limited to moderate evidence that there is at least an analgesic effect for mid-portion Achilles tendinopathies for both the short and long-term. There is conflicting evidence about tendon tissue healing and long-term function. All studies examined the mid-portion of the tendon.

PT Limited evidence there is no effect of GTN on patellar tendinopathy up to six months.

LET Limited to moderate evidence that there is at least an analgesic effect for LET.

RCT Weak to limited evidence of a short-term analgesic effect on RCT tendon issues, with one study having a high risk of bias. The short-term analgesic effect was not as strong as corticosteroids. There is limited evidence that no significant, long-term changes occur from GTN on rotator cuff tendinopathies.

Items to Note

One review found there to be a better response to chronic over acute tendinopathy for Achilles, lateral elbow, and shoulder tendon injuries. Multiple reviews state there is a better effect on pain and function when GTN is added to an eccentric loading program.

Final recommendation

GTN is a promising intervention that warrants more research regarding its potential healing properties. It seems to have at least a short-term pain-relieving effect, with a questionable effect on long-term tendon healing and function. One major adverse effect stated in virtually all of the research is that GTN can cause headaches, up to a strong enough degree that patients need to stop treatment.

It is our determination that GTN can be used in conjunction with eccentric loading protocols for an analgesic effect, with the possibility of increased function. However, the potential for headaches should cause one to take caution, particularly if they have a problematic medical history in that area.

Pain Medication

Medication is one of the most frequently used interventions for pain related to many diagnoses, including tendinopathies. This section will focus on the major drug type used for pain relief, non-steroidal anti-inflammatory drugs, or NSAIDs for short. *NSAIDs* are taken orally and are available over-the-counter or as prescribed by a medical doctor. They block specific enzymes in the body that would normally produce inflammatory markers to signal the body to feel pain. The most commonly used NSAIDs are aspirin, ibuprofen (ex: Advil, Motrin), and naproxen (ex: Aleve).

Pros	Cons
• convenient, relatively cost-effective and easy to use	• there is a potential for dependence and abuse • consistent, long-term use can cause gastro-intestinal issues, kidney damage, and high blood pressure

Tendon-specific Research

LET　　Limited evidence shows NSAIDs were as effective in pain and function for LET at less than three months compared to corticosteroid injections. However, neither intervention was found to be significantly effective for the long-term.

RCT　　Limited evidence shows NSAIDs are effective for both pain and function for RCT issues, but not significantly effective for the long-term.

Items to Note

Given that tendinopathy is primarily a non-inflammatory proliferative disorder, both NSAIDs and other pain relievers like paracetamol (ex: Tylenol, acetaminophen) would have limited effect except for pain relief and possible negative effects on collagen synthesis in the long run. The only possible functional benefits of NSAIDs (over non-NSAID pain medications) may be if there are issues with other inflammation in the paratendon areas (surrounding the tendon) or compressive loading areas (insertional Achilles or rotator cuff tendinopathy) which may also be aggravated at the same time as the tendinopathy.

Final recommendation

Pain medication is clearly effective at decreasing pain associated with tendon issues, particularly in the short term. However, because of the potential adverse effects that can be experienced with long-term use, we recommend only using medication for short-term pain management while seeking other treatment. The most common medications sold and prescribed essentially only mask one's pain; they do not promote healing or counteract tendon degradation. Consult your doctor or physical therapist to determine if you should use medication for your particular type of tendinopathy (even if the medication is available over-the-counter). This is especially necessary if you suspect you have chronic pain symptoms because you could end up taking the medication for an extended period of time, thus opening the door to potential adverse effects like dependency.

Stretching Exercises

Stretching exercises are used to increase range of motion and are conventionally thought of as beneficial for joint mobility, as well as relieving muscle pain and tightness. Stretching can be divided into three types: static, dynamic, and ballistic. Static stretching involves long positional holds and is what is most imagined when the term is used. Dynamic stretching involves quick bursts of stretching that are performed repeatedly over one or more joints. Ballistic stretching is explosive in nature and used in sport-specific instances like high kicks or split kicks for martial artists. This type of stretching is not recommended for any type of injury.

Pros	Cons
• cost-effective, short-term tension and pain relief, improves mobility	• can be time-consuming • can aggravate pain if performed too frequently or forcefully

Tendon-specific Research

AT	Achilles pain and stiffness recommendations, though based on weak evidence, state that bent and straight-knee calf stretching can reduce pain and improve patient satisfaction for those with impaired dorsiflexion. Both static and dynamic stretching may have benefits in a complementary manner for Achilles issues. Stretching alone does not seem to have as significant of an effect for Achilles tendon injuries, as does stretching added to strengthening exercises.
PT	Stretching alone does not seem to have as great of an effect on patellar tendon injuries, as does stretching added to strengthening exercises.
LET/MET	Stretching alone does not seem to have as great of an effect on elbow tendon injuries, as does stretching added to strengthening exercises. Limited evidence states there is not a significant difference between stretching and strengthening for the elbow.
RCT	May have benefits when coupled with other interventions like exercise and manual therapy.

Items to Note

Dynamic stretching may have a better effect than static in regard to pain relief and function. Dynamic stretching can be seen in a more similar vein than passive in regards to eccentrics, and thus more effective on the tendon. There is weak evidence that shows little difference between stretching and strengthening in all outcomes and tendon areas. There is a surprising lack of research that specifically addresses stretching and tendon injuries.

Final recommendation

Stretching appears to have a small positive effect on tendon injury, particularly when there is limited range of motion and/or it is paired with complementary interventions like eccentric exercise training and manual therapy. Static stretching alone does not appear to have a significant effect on pain or function. We recommend both static and dynamic stretching as part of a rehabilitation routine that focuses on strengthening exercises and other pain-relieving interventions.

Supplements

Supplements are dietary additives that are meant to enhance the body's mechanisms but are not considered food. There is a wide array of supplements available for consumption. Some of these have been theorized to improve tendon function, such as glucosamine, antioxidants, vitamin C and collagen, hyaluronic acid, and others.

Pros	Cons
• easily attainable, cost-effective	• possible adverse health reactions if taken incorrectly or if supplements are untested/ unregulated

Tendon-specific Research

PT Very limited evidence from a single trial shows a mild positive effect with fatty acids and antioxidants. Results should be taken with a grain of salt as only one study has been performed.

LET Same as above

RCT Limited evidence from two trials show a mild positive effect with fatty acids and antioxidants.

OTHER Cursory research *in vitro* (in the lab) on human tendon cells, and in lab rats, suggests that vitamin C and collagen may help increase collagen synthesis rates in tendons. There are similar results in rats for hyaluronic acid and glucosamine chondroitin. These supplements tend to show greater effects for lacerated, torn, or ruptured tendons and little to no effect in tendinopathies in lab rats.

Items to Note

There are many different types of supplements used for medical and nutritional purposes. Many of these have not been properly studied for how they interact with other supplements, not to mention prescription drugs. Research results are very heterogeneous and should be taken with a grain of salt. Other supplements like BPC 157 have not been studied.

Final Recommendation

Although there is potential scientific mechanism and positive lab results for certain researched supplements, we do not recommend supplement usage as an intervention for tendon issues at this time. The research in this area is weak, limited, and contains too many heterogeneous variables. The benefits for tendon issues is promising but not significant enough to endorse. There are also many unknowns as to interactions that may occur when supplements are mixed with other supplements and/or medications.

Additional Vitamin C and Gelatin Supplement Commentary

Those with disposable income may want to experiment with supplements, but those on a budget can certainly get by without them, as there are other options available. If you do choose to purchase supplements, those available at most stores are sufficient. Don't waste your money on expensive collagen supplements that claim to benefit specific tendons or ligaments. Consult your doctor and/or physical therapist before beginning a supplement regimen. Most of the anecdotal evidence in athletes seems to suggest a dose of vitamin C-enriched gelatin before a rehabilitation session may improve collagen synthesis over placebo.

Research by Melendez-Hevia et al shows that glycine is potentially the limiting amino acid in collagen synthesis:

> Detailed assessment of all possible sources of glycine shows that synthesis from serine accounts for more than 85 percent of the total, and that the amount of glycine available from synthesis (about 3 grams per day) together with that available from the diet (in the range of 1.5 to 3 grams per day) may fall significantly short of the amount needed for all metabolic uses, including collagen synthesis, by about 10 grams per day for a 70-kilogram human.

Substituting other protein sources (such as whey and soy) would be inferior. Per a different study, whey and soy protein only have about 0.6 grams of glycine per serving (1.8 grams per 100 grams of whey, or 2.6 grams per 100 grams of soy—about 2 percent of each), while the amino acid content of collagen and gelatin is approximately 26 percent of glycine. The usual supplement weight of collagen in most studies is 15 grams, so one would be effectively getting approximately 3.75 grams of glycine per 15-gram supplemental collagen/gelatin intake. Supplementing glycine or collagen (which is rich in glycine) can possibly overcome rate-limiting steps while comparative protein sources will not.

Since the rate-limiting step proposed by Melendez-Hevia et al is 10 grams per day and the body can produce 3 grams through synthesis with another 1.5-3 grams available from the diet (per their results, this presents a deficit of approximately 4-5.5 grams. Thus, we would suggest the proper collagen intake be around 20-25 grams per day in order to obtain another 5.5 grams (roughly) of glycine, coupled with the body's natural production and dietary intake to match the 10-gram rate-limiting reaction. We are unsure if this collagen should be taken in a single 20-25-gram dosage, two doses of 10-12.5 grams, or even three doses of a lesser amount. What we can affirm is at least one dose should be taken before a rehabilitation session is performed.

It should also be noted that this is not enough data to determine if this method will increase collagen synthesis to the point that an objective difference is made in the long run. More studies are needed to confirm if this is true. It could potentially be a placebo effect, or small gains that add up to an insignificant result. All this being said, early research seems to be promising.

In conclusion, supplements probably won't hurt and they could help. Those with disposable income may want to utilize them, but if you are on a budget they are not necessary as the gains will be marginally better at most. Be wary of expensive supplements that claim to benefit specific tendons or ligaments. We would recommend avoiding these altogether.

Transcutaneous Electrical Nerve Stimulation (TENS)

Transcutaneous electrical nerve stimulation (TENS) is generally used as a therapeutic intervention to decrease pain. TENS uses a device that delivers an electrical current via pads that are attached to the skin at or near the site of injury. Different settings can be adjusted to deliver electrical charge that stimulates nerves for sensation using the same device. The device can be adjusted for frequency, intensity, and pulse width depending on the type of response desired for a specific diagnosis.

Pros	Cons
• relatively safe, inexpensive • can be used at home if proper education is given • has versatility of utilization for a variety of health issues	• can cause skin irritation • should not be used in sensitive areas like the eyes, or over metal implants/pacemakers • can cause unwanted pain and nerve irritation if turned up too high

Tendon-specific Research

AT   Weak evidence that TENS can have a positive effect on Achilles tendinosis when using the burst setting.

LET   Evidence is currently too conflicting.

RCT   Evidence is currently too poor to suggest an effect.

Items to Note

One can increase the intensity on the device that delivers TENS to the point that it can stimulate motor nerves and cause a muscle contraction. This is not the intention when using the term TENS. When an electrical current is used to cause a muscle contraction, it is referred to as *neuromuscular electrical stimulation* (NMES). This is used for strengthening.

Final Recommendation

There is very little evidence available about the relationship between TENS and tendon issues. Much of the published research discusses TENS being used to treat other conditions associated with pain, and chronic pain relief in general. While TENS does have a generally favorable effect on pain, it does not seem to be as effective as other therapeutic options for tendon issues. After reviewing the available research, we believe it is an intervention that has the ability to mask pain but does not necessarily promote tendon healing. We recommend TENS for short-term pain relief; however, we recommend more reliable, well-established treatment techniques for long-term care.

Wait and see (AKA watchful waiting)

The "wait and see" (or *watchful waiting*) approach involves the patient not actively applying an intervention to the area of injury. Instead, they seek to rest and see what happens—whether the pain will resolve itself through normal daily movement. This act of resting is, in itself, the intervention.

There is some debate as to how to define this as an intervention and whether repetitive overuse movements should still be modified to reduce the potential pain source.

Pros	Cons
• cost-effective • requires no additional time or energy	• can take a long time for pain to resolve, while one has to cope with the pain/dysfunction at least in the short-term • might have to adapt function and movement to allow for needed rest

Tendon-specific Research

LET This approach may, ultimately, have a similar long-term effect for pain relief as CST injections. There is some evidence that there is little difference between general, non-surgical interventions and the wait and see approach, but it is possible that this is due to activity modification and education. This conflicts with other research, which shows the addition of eccentric exercises is more beneficial for LET than wait and see.

RCT Limited evidence to suggest a "wait and see" approach may have similar outcomes to CST injections in both the intermediate and long-term.

Items to Note

The "wait and see" approach has been poorly defined in the research and there is no set standard of how to measure it when it is included as an intervention in a clinical trial. It is often unclear if education and medical advice is included when this method is used as an intervention, as well as if activities were modified or avoided altogether. For this reason, the results of these studies should be taken with a grain of salt. There is also an issue with a lack of distinguishing between acute tendon pain and chronic pain. The former may resolve with a generalized wait and see approach, but this would probably not be the case in cases where the pain is chronic.

Final Recommendation

A "wait and see" approach may be as beneficial as other recommended interventions for LET (lateral elbow) or MET (medial elbow) issues likely only in situations involving acute tendon pain. We still recommend seeking guidance from a medical provider about activity modifications and pain relief options while waiting. For all other tendon areas, we would not recommend this approach over other supported interventions due to conflicting/weak evidence.

Calcific Tendinopathy

Calcific Tendinopathy is a different variation of tendinopathy from the most common forms. Thus, it is present in very little scientific literature. Calcific tendinopathies involve calcifications physically forming in the tendon and muscle tissue, which causes pain and mobility issues. This calcification process occurs most often in the rotator cuff of the shoulder, especially in the supraspinatus tendon. The specific pathophysiology as to why this happens is still relatively unknown, but the most likely theories involve limited vascularity in this area, coupled with metabolic changes and overuse.

Since calcific tendinopathy can have a more severe pain presentation, the most effective treatments proposed in the literature we examined focused first on short-term, non-invasive pain-relieving techniques before progressing to more functionally-based exercise and loading protocols. Here are some noteworthy suggestions we came across:

- High-energy *extracorporeal shockwave therapy* (ECST) has a more favorable potential benefit than other passive modalities. Thus, could be considered early on in treatment. Radial ECST and ultrasound guided needling are also potential options.

- One or two corticosteroid injections for pain management seems to be a well-supported short-term option.

- Ultrasound guided lavage is a newer, but promising, intervention that may compare favorably to ECST. However, this is based on low-quality evidence; more high-quality, randomized trials are needed to confirm this.

These interventions should be considered after more conservative treatment options fail. Even then, they would typically be performed in conjunction with more conservative treatments in order to effectively break up the calcium deposits.

According to the Elshewy review, the disease progresses in formative and resorptive phases. If the patient can tolerate the pain through the resorptive phases the condition will normally resolve on its own. If conservative treatment and alternatives to conservative treatment fail after 6+ months (though preferably 12+) due to function and pain not improving significantly, surgical intervention to remove the calcific deposits is a last resort and carries with it the potential for complications and longer rehabilitation times. For the shoulder, the best option is arthroscopic removal.

Bracing

Regarding bracing for tendinopathy, we did not find much in the scientific literature. The gold standard article mentioned in the first chapter of this book, *Achilles Pain, Stiffness, and Muscle Power Deficits; Midportion Achilles Tendinopathy Revision*, suggests that several interventions should not be used at this time:

- Heel Lifts (Evidence Level D) — The research is conflicting, so no recommendation can be made.
- Orthoses (Evidence Level D) — The research is conflicting, so no recommendation can be made.
- Night Splints (Evidence Level C) — Weak evidence that night splints should not be used.

Other interventions, such as taping, suggest expert opinion (Evidence Level F) that elastic taping should not be used, but rigid taping can be used to decrease the strain on the tendon.

Unfortunately, the other types of bracing, such as elbow or patellar bands, do not have much, if any, research based on our observations. These bands are usually one to two inches in width and tighten when positioned at or just below the knee or elbow, on the painful tendon, and compressed to alleviate pain. These band braces should not to be confused with compression sleeves, which are typically six to twelve inches in length and extend far above and below the tendon. Compression sleeves are not effective for tendinopathy, though they can help keep the tendon area warm if it gets stiff easily.

From anecdotal experience with climbers, the elbow band can relieve pain and allow a patient to continue to maintain their sport-specific activity while performing rehabilitation exercise on the side. Therefore, at this juncture, we would rate it at Evidence Level F, to be performed at clinician and patient discretion, in conjunction with rehabilitation exercises.

Pain Neuroscience Education Talking Points

GENERAL INFORMATION ABOUT PAIN

- Pain is an alarm system to send threat signals from the body to the brain and back (Butler & Mosely: Explain Pain book). This system can behave strangely or break down entirely for unknown reasons. This system can also be amplified by environmental influences like stress, unhealthy habits, and life events.

- Imaging studies (ex: ultrasound and MRI) of various tissues such as the back and tendons often show there are signs of degeneration in healthy populations. This "degeneration" is asymptomatic, which means it does not cause any pain or decreased function in the people who have it (Chapter 2, Tendinopathy, Rehabilitation, and Outcomes section). In other words, even if a tissue is "damaged" on imaging does not mean it can't retain good function without pain or that it is incapable of being rehabilitated to a state of good function without pain.

- The farther out from a specific acute injury the pain persists, the more likely the involvement of scenarios involving chronic pain (Chapter 5, Pain Education section). The most common time is about 3+ months.

- "Even though evidence supports the reduction of pain over time with the utilization of PNE (pain neuroscience education), a sudden, total resolution of pain is biologically questionable. The concept of reconceptualizing pain, a cornerstone of PNE, aims to have patients see their pain differently. This implies that even though they still experience pain, they think differently about it, equating it to sensitization of the nervous system versus the health of the tissues. Furthermore, this reconceptualization imparts a message of "despite the pain," it is worthwhile to move, exercise, engage, and continue in daily activities and not necessary to seek additional care for the sensitization (pain). This behavior change is the key to changing any patient's healthcare status, that is, smoking, weight gain, etc." (Louw study, The efficacy of pain neuroscience education on musculoskeletal pain: A systematic review of the literature).

- The majority of studies still do not know what causes all of the factors involving tendinopathy pain (Chapter 5, Tendinopathy Pain).

AGGRAVATING EXERCISES VS. PAINFUL EXERCISES

In the clinic, we tend to educate patients to avoid "aggravating exercises" rather than avoiding "painful exercises."

- Some exercises may cause pain, but they improve the performance and function of the injured area(s) after the exercise and/or by the next session. For example, think about rehabilitation exercises: they may cause pain during a session, but the pain is often the same or decreases over time with subsequent sessions.

- Some exercises may not cause pain, but they make the injury worse over time in terms of both pain and function. For instance, if an athlete has tendinopathy with pain and slightly decreased function, but they are able to warmup in a particular session of their sport where the pain goes away they think they can practice or train fully on it. However, after the practice or training session, several hours later and by the next session the symptoms and functions continue to get worse. This is one of the most common scenarios where non-painful exercises or training may still be aggravating the tendon via overload of intensity and volume.

- Some exercises may be both painful and aggravating leading to both increased pain and decreased performance. This is most common with acute injuries.

TENDINOPATHY PAIN

ACUTE PAIN

- Isometrics (ex: contracting a muscle without the muscle lengthening or shortening) can be used in 3 different ways:
  - For use in athletes to help decrease pain while maintaining volume of sport-specific activities during competition seasons.
  - For pain relief prior to eccentric-concentric or heavy-slow resistance interventions in rehabilitation, especially if they are having difficulty or poor control performing the rehabilitation exercises due to pain.
  - Isometrics can be performed multiple times throughout the day to reduce pain, even on non-rehabilitation days.
- The total volume of isometric pain-reduction intervention holds ranges from 3-4 minutes, based on studies that used 5 sets of 45 seconds (3:45 total), 6 sets of 40 seconds (4:00 total), and 24 sets of 10 seconds (4:00 total) at a weight of 70-85% 1 RM (or about 6-12 RM). We tend to prefer less sets and longer amounts of time, but you can modify accordingly based on what works best for you and/or your patient.
- This principle is for acute pain cases. Pain may be grounded to a numerical scale in the no pain to light pain range (0 to 1-3 range) as opposed to moderate to intense to highest pain range (4-6 to 7-9 to 10) to indicate safe versus non-safe training intensities (Mascaro's systematic graded approach). Other assessment factors such as improvement of function and pain across several rehabilitation sessions should be used to test the scale against to ensure that rehabilitation is progressing in the right direction.
- Alternative exercises to reduce pain and improve tendon function and loading should be considered, especially if pain is too severe. For instance, with biceps tendinopathy, if supinated curls are too painful, hammer or pronated curls may be the most useful rehabilitation exercises to start with. As load tolerance increases, usually the pain will also decrease too. Eventually, supinated curls may be integrated.
- Pain typically resolves gradually as the rehabilitation program progresses through the various stages, which include: isometric work, strength, functional strength, speed, plyometrics, and back to full level of activity or sport. If the pain is not resolving gradually, but function is continuing to improve through the various stages, and it has been longer than 3+ months you may be dealing with a chronic case.

CHRONIC PAIN

- Ensure the patient is properly educated on all of the talking points above.
- While pain rarely resolves suddenly, chronic pain can lessen over time and completely resolve in some cases.
- Most of the pain interventions in the conservative adjuncts and non-conservative adjuncts will NOT be helpful scenarios involving chronic pain. Please discuss with your doctor and/or physical therapist for more details.
- Use systematic, graded exposure to increase any exercise tolerance. For instance, if walking causes Achilles or knee pain, begin with 5 minutes of walking and slowly increase by no more than a minute or two each session. You may even desire to only increase the time every other session. Focus on slow, gradual improvements.
- Encourage the patient to participate in exercise and enjoyable activities with friends and family that do not increase their level of pain. Pain is not indicative of tissue damage. Movement and getting back into an enjoyable daily routine is good for the healing process.

- Have the patient engage in novel movements that do not cause pain. Novel movements indicate to the nervous system that the movement of specific areas (or tendons, in this case) is not a threat. This helps to decrease the sensitization that has occurred with the movements that accumulated to cause chronic pain in the first place.

- Other strategies may include increasing "relaxation" activities like meditation, massage, deep breathing, and other things that decrease stress and relax the body. These can help to decrease the sensitization of the nervous system, which may positively influence chronic pain.

- Some other avenues to explore are Cognitive Behavioral Therapy (CBT) and sensory discrimination training.

BOTH CHRONIC AND ACUTE

- Some flare-ups of pain and other symptoms are a normal part of the rehabilitation process. If the rehabilitation loading program is gradual and progressive, there is little reason to make changes aside from repeating a session a time or two. If the flare-up is because something changed drastically (ex: adding exercises, lots of different intensities or volume, returning to a sport), the clinician should examine the program to see if any modifications should be made.

- Rehabilitation is a gradual process and should not be rushed. The greatest predictor of injuries are previous injuries. Also, one of the easiest ways to end up with chronic pain is to continue to push through acute painful exercises and activities, as many athletes and workers are prone to do.

GOLD STANDARD:
ECCENTRIC-CONCENTRIC LOADING PROGRAM + ISOMETRICS FOR PAIN

Clinicians should look to identify and modify programs based on several criteria:

- Consider whether the tendon is low or high reactivity and modify loading interventions based on how the tendon responds to loading

- Consider if the pain is acute or chronic and provide adequate pain education

- Stage the tendon (reactive/dysrepair and degenerative) and apply appropriate interventions

- Apply appropriate pain interventions

- Correct and modify any technique compensations due to pain

- Correct any weakness, instability, lack of control, and deficits in range of motion (ROM) with movement at the joint and including joints proximal and distal to the affected tendon

- Consider intrinsic and extrinsic factors that increase propensity for injury, reinjury, and aggravation

POSSIBLE ADJUNCTS TO THE GOLD STANDARD:

LIKELY TO HELP	MAY HELP	UNLIKELY/DON'T USE
• Manual Therapy (small effect?)	• Iontophoresis (acute/reactive only)	• Wait and See
• Stretching (if limited ROM)	• TENS (short-term pain)	• Supplements (research sparse)
• Pain Medications (short-term pain)	• Ergonomics (clinician discretion)	• Ultrasound

Most adjuncts to the gold standard of treatment only help under specific conditions (limited range of motion, in acute/reactive tendons, or with short-term pain) which is why they must be paired with eccentric-concentric loading programs to build up strength and load tolerance.

IF CONSERVATIVE TREATMENT FAILS

NON-CONSERVATIVE ADJUNCTS

After conservative treatment has failed, some interventions can be considered to possibly be helpful **in conjunction with more conservative treatment**. Most of these interventions do not promote any tendon healing or increased load tolerance of the tendon and provide only pain relief. The research around many of these is either conflicting or sparse and only show mild benefits at most. Approach with caution.

LIKELY TO HELP	MAY HELP	UNLIKELY/DON'T USE
• ECST (small positive effect but research may be biased; possibly better for calcific)	• Needling (short-term pain)	• PRP/ABI/Prolo (very conflicting research showing small positive to no results; promising in the research with tendon tears but not tendinopathy)
• Nitro (short-term pain and possible functional improvement but possible severe side effects like headaches)	• LLLT (short-term pain at certain wavelengths)	
	• CST injections (short-term pain, no more than 1-2 injections)	
	• Botox (Upper extremity)	

Due to the scarcity or conflicting research with many of these non-conservative adjuncts, some physical therapists recommend avoiding them altogether. Isometrics seem to be the gold standard for acute pain relief at the current juncture, and chronic pain is unlikely to be resolved by these interventions. Effective pain neuroscience education paired with movement is likely to be more helpful in the long run. Again, a high amount of caution and second opinions should be used if these interventions are being considered.

IF CONSERVATIVE TREATMENT (12+ MONTHS) &
NON-CONSERVATIVE ADJUNCTS FAIL

LAST RESORT

Surgery (~75% success rate for Achilles. Other areas have more variable success rates, and side effects can be common.)

SUMMARY OF TENDINOPATHY REHABILITATION RECOMMENDATIONS

Chapter 6 was exceptionally long and detailed, so a summary is necessary.

Ordering of a sample rehabilitation session.

1. **Warm-up and mobility**: Mobility and very light stretching especially if the tendon is stiff to warm up. Heat can be added in this section to help warm up the surrounding tissues if they are exceptionally stiff and painful.

2. **Skilled techniques**: Soft tissue work such as massage, manual therapy, or mobilization at clinician's discretion. Neuromuscular training to focus on good movement patterns, if any.

3. **Pain management**: Isometrics to reduce pain for the tendon loading program. Heat and possibly analgesics can be used too. Can be done prior to warm up and skilled techniques if necessary.

4. **Targeted eccentric-concentric exercises**: For golfer's elbow wrist curls, for tennis elbow reverse wrist curls, for biceps tendinopathy biceps curls, for patellar decline board squats, etc. If a patient is further along in rehabilitation, compound exercises and sports specific movements or occupational tasks can be added.

5. **Peripheral strength/endurance or other kinetic chain exercises**: This can include strengthening antagonists to make sure there is adequate ratios of strength and strengthening the muscles proximal and distal to the joint. If there is a lack of control, stability, or weakness above and below the joint(s) where the tendinopathy is that can be placed here too.

6. **Flexibility and any follow up mobility work**: Mobility following flexibility can help sustain it if there is new range of motion from the flexibility work. Some prefer flexibility before strength work which can also work as long as it doesn't interfere with the strength training.

The following parameters for eccentric-concentric rehabilitation training.

- **Intensity**—We recommend approximately 6-12 sets with about 10-15 repetitions per set every 2 days (average of about 60 to 180 repetitions per 2-day rehabilitation session) or a total volume of about 21-42 sets per week based on the current research.

- **Frequency**—We recommend starting with 3x per week eccentric-concentric strength training and modifying from there based on how the patient presents and according to the intensity and volume recommendations as needed. The benefits of less frequency per week on improving patient compliance and possible synergy with the collagen synthesis rates and helpfulness with highly irritable tendons makes this a good choice.

- **Tempo**—We recommend for the initial phases of rehabilitation an eccentric of 2-3s and a controlled concentric phase of about 1-2s. This would be approximately 3010 or 2010 or 3020 or 2020 tempo. This can be modified depending on how a patient is presenting such as if they need rest between repetitions or depending on the stage of the rehabilitation. If a patient or athlete is progressing in their rehabilitation well, a faster eccentric and concentric portion may be necessary to start preparing them for the explosive and plyometric nature of many sports.
- **Alternative protocol**—1 to 2 exercises at 3 sets per exercises for 30 to 50 repetitions per set. 2-3 second eccentric and 1s concentric, depending on how the tendon is presenting and time constraints (3010 or 2010 tempo). Stay 3-5 repetitions short of failure, at least to start. This lowers the chance of reinjury. Can be performed with pain if the pain does not increase afterward or by the next session and function is improving. Progress by 1-3 reps per session. Once you hit 50 repetitions, up the weight and drop down to 30 repetitions. As the tendinopathy starts to improve, drop to 30 repetitions after a 50 repetition set and slowly work down into the 25, 20, 15, and 10 repetition range by 2-5 reps per couple sessions while slowly increasing the weight and staying a couple repetitions short of failure.

Rehabilitation stages

1. Reduce pain and irritability
2. Improve strength
3. Improve functional strength
4. Increase power
5. Develop stretch shorten cycle return to sport

Overall, for the pain and irritability stage.

Determining the stage of the tendinopathy is important. Reactive or dysrepair, reactive-on-degenerative, or degenerative. This will inform much of the rehab later.

- Clinicians must first distinguish whether the pain is acute or chronic or more likely to be one or the other. Proper pain neuroscience education (PNE) must be given accordingly to ensure that the patient has a proper understanding of their pain and is not going to make it worse by catastrophizing it or thinking that they are doing damage if it is chronic.
- Clinicians should look at a patient's daily life, work, and/or sport in order to recommend removing any aggravating exercises if the tendinopathy is being made worse by overuse. Also, remove any exercises that put compressive loading or high tension on the tendon as they have the possibility to aggravate or re-aggravate the tendon increasing pain and irritability.
- Use isometrics to reduce pain. 3-4 minutes of total isometric tension at 70-80% MCIV from 3-24 sets. Typically, sets of 1 minute or 45s are probably the least tedious. Can be done multiple times throughout the day as needed.
- Anti-inflammatory use such as NSAIDs in this stage can be used to reduce pain. Though they may decrease collagen synthesis, you're not introducing exercises for rehabilitation of the tendon at this juncture. Anti-inflammatories may help if there is minimal inflammation (as opposed to none in many cases) or associated surrounding structural inflammation such as paratendonitis, especially in compressed areas like the rotator cuff, infrapatellar area, or Achilles insertion area.
- Other modalities like heat that can reduce pain can be helpful. Some evidence has shown that dexamethasone in reactive tendons helps to calm them down.

- Light stretching if there is a reduction in range of motion at the joints
- A skilled medical professional such as a physical therapist can look for weaknesses or compensations at the joints above, at, and below the affected area(s) as well as prescribe exercises to start working on them.

Overall, for the improve strength stage.

1. Continue isometrics if pain is an issue. Continue to educate on PNE if you suspect the patient is having doubts because their pain level is staying constant or not reducing as fast as they think it should.
2. Don't progress exercises too fast especially coming off reactive or highly irritable tendons. Progression does not have to be every session but every 2-3 sessions if it's responding to rehabilitation slower.
3. Stick with simple progressions for improving strength are adding light weights (going from 2 lbs to 3 lbs to 4 lbs and so on) or resistance bands (going from the easiest to a slightly more difficult one to a slightly more difficult one) if you are using isolation exercises. These are the most common ones you'll see. Some other small common ones are addition repetitions such as going from 10 reps to 11 reps to 12 reps over subsequent 1-3 workouts as tolerated. Another one is to add in an additional set at not to failure repetitions. For example, if you're doing 3 sets of 10 repetitions then you may add in another set at 1-3 repetitions and slowly add in volume to that set over subsequent workouts if you lack the ability for minimal resistance increase.
4. Use slow to moderate speed during the repetitions, both eccentric and concentric phases. Generally, 2010 or 3010 is a good place to start.
5. Aim to slowly increase the progression, typically by load but alternatives such as repetitions or sets can work if it's difficult to increase the load or the reactivity is starting to come back because of the load.
6. Make sure you are addressing the kinetic chain above and below the area of tendinopathy too!

Overall, for the improve functional strength stage.

1. Continue isometrics for pain if needed.
2. Do not progress too fast.
3. Generally, prior rehabilitation exercises that are easier may be removed and substituted out at this point if needed.
4. Addition of compound exercises should be looked at closely for any signs of compensations and application to strengthening kinetic chain.
5. Slowly add in these functional exercises as volume. If the volume seems to be too much, clinicians can reduce the isolation exercises in favor of some compound movements. For instance, going with 1-2 sets for the isolation exercises after the compound movements are added.

Overall, for the power stage.

1. Start with mid-range power work before moving to more end range to avoid compressive loads on the tendon.
2. Continue to track pain and function post-workouts and the day after to ensure that you aren't increasing progression too fast. If the tendon starts to get irritable again, have a back off plan.
3. If power is not needed such as in some sedentary patients or active workers, start to introduce task related activities in conjunction with strategies to avoid overuse

4. Make sure you are addressing the kinetic chain above and below the area of tendinopathy too!

Overall, for the power stage and return to sport.

1. If your medical practitioner such as a doctor or physical therapist is not as familiar with these exercises, this is where consulting a sports doctor or physical therapist or other professional (athletic trainer, CSCS, coach, or whoever runs these activities for sports or sports teams) in order to get a good progression reintroducing these exercises back into the athlete's regimen.

2. From our experience, most lay people and athletes who have not trained any type of explosiveness or plyometric regimens jump into them far too fast. Depth drops or rebounds tend to be done with a height that is way too high and too many repetitions. Start with a very small amount and not to failure. Increase the volume slowly over time along with adding in faster and faster sports specific movements.

Overall, for continuing sport specific activities with an injury.

1. Consult with the appropriate medical professionals with any injury.

2. One general rule of thumb is if you get injured, make an appointment with the appropriate medical professional right away. There's usually a lag time of couple weeks getting an appointment, so if it's a moderate to severe injury, you want to get in as quickly as possible. If it's a minor injury that "heals" and you don't want professional help (usually not a good idea still), you can always cancel the appointment later if need.

3. Please consult with the appropriate medical professionals. Look for doctors, physical therapists, trainers, and ones like these who work with athletes if you're trying to get back to playing sports or activities at a high level. Finding out who local sports teams or universities use for their athletes can usually work well.

4. Generally, continue with your training regimen with the exercises away from the injury (e.g. if it's golfer's elbow, continue with all lower body and core work). Exercises around the injury can usually be continued if they do not aggravate it and make it worse in pain and function.

Additionally, Acute:Chronic workload ratio (ACWR) and Heart Rate Variability can be two scientifically based protocols to use for coaches, athletes, and/or medical professionals in order to help prevent injury and reinjury. There is limited but positive research in this area especially in the arena of preventing injury, which should be transferable to anyone rehabilitating from injury as well.

NOTES

1   *The Centre for Evidence-Based Medicine develops, promotes and disseminates better evidence for healthcare.* Centre for Evidence-Based Medicine. 15 1 2019. www.cebm.net

2   *Published Guidelines.* Academy of Orthopaedic Physical Therapy. 15 1 2019. www.orthopt.org/content/practice/clinical -practice-guidelines addendum for mid-portion Achilles: https://www.jospt.org/doi/pdfplus/10.2519/jospt.2018.0302

3   Kaeding C, Best TM. *Tendinosis: Pathophysiology and Nonoperative Treatment.* Sports Health. 2009 Jul; 1(4): 284–292. https://www.ncbi.nlm.nih.gov/pmc/articles/PMC3445129/

4   Khan KM, Cook JL, Bonar F, Harcourt P, Astrom M. *Histopathology of common tendinopathies. Update and implications for clinical management.* Sports Med. 1999 Jun;27(6):393-408. https://www.ncbi.nlm.nih.gov/pubmed/10418074

5   Khan KM, Cook JL, Kannus P, Maffulli N, Bonar SF. *Time to abandon the "tendonitis" myth.* BMJ. 2002 Mar 16;324(7338):626-7. https://www.ncbi.nlm.nih.gov/pmc/articles/pmid/11895810/

6   Maffulli N, Khan KM, Puddu G. *Overuse tendon conditions: time to change a confusing terminology.* Arthroscopy. 1998; 14: 840– 843. http://dx.doi.org/10.1016/s0749-8063(98)70021-0

7   Almekinders LC. *Tendonitis and other chronic tendinopathies.* J Am Acad Orthop Surg. 1998 May-Jun;6(3):157-64. https:// www.ncbi.nlm.nih.gov/pubmed/9682077

8   Scott A, Squier K, Alfredson H. *ICON 2019: International Scientific Tendinopathy Symposium Consensus: Clinical Terminology.* Br J Sports Med. 2019 Aug 9. pii: bjsports-2019-100885. doi: 10.1136/bjsports-2019-100885. [Epub ahead of print]. https://www.ncbi.nlm.nih.gov/pubmed/31399426

9   Nagrale AV, Herd CR, Ganvir S, et al. *Cyriax physiotherapy versus phonophoresis with supervised exercise in subjects with lateral epicondylalgia: a randomized clinical trial.* J Man Manip Ther 2009;17:171–8. https://www.ncbi.nlm.nih.gov/pmc/articles /PMC2762836/

10 Arnoczky SP, Lavagnino M, Egerbacher M. *The mechanobiological aetiopathogenesis of tendinopathy: is it the over-stimulation or the under-stimulation of tendon cells?* Int J Exp Pathol. 2007 Aug; 88(4): 217–226. https://www.ncbi.nlm.nih.gov/pmc /articles/PMC2517314/

11 Abate M, Gravare-Silbernagel K, Siljeholm C, Di Iorio A, De Amicis D, Salini V, Werner S, Paganelli R. *Pathogenesis of tendinopathies: inflammation or degeneration?* Arthritis Res Ther. 2009; 11(3): 235. https://www.ncbi.nlm.nih.gov/pmc/articles /PMC2714139/

12 Cook JL, Purdam CR. *Is tendon pathology a continuum? A pathology model to explain the clinical presentation of load-induced tendinopathy.* Send to Br J Sports Med. 2009 Jun;43(6):409-16. doi: 10.1136/bjsm.2008.051193. Epub 2008 Sep 23. https:// www.ncbi.nlm.nih.gov/pubmed/18812414

13 Fu SC, Rolf C, Cheuk, YC, Lui PPY, Chan KM. *Deciphering the pathogenesis of tendinopathy: a three-stages process.* Sports Med Arthrosc Rehabil Ther Technol. 2010; 2: 30. https://www.ncbi.nlm.nih.gov/pmc/articles/PMC3006368/

14 J L Cook, E Rio, C R Purdam, S I Docking. *Revisiting the continuum model of tendon pathology: what is its merit in clinical practice and research?* Br J Sports Med. 2016 Oct; 50(19): 1187–1191. https://www.ncbi.nlm.nih.gov/pmc/articles/PMC5118437/

15 Hodgson RJ, O'Connor PJ, Grainger AJ. *Tendon and ligament imaging.* Br J Radiol. 2012 Aug; 85(1016): 1157–1172. https://www.ncbi.nlm.nih.gov/pmc/articles/PMC3495576/

16 Longo UG, Ronga M, Maffulli N. *Achilles tendinopathy.* Sports Med Arthrosc Rev. 2009 Jun;17(2):112-26. https://www.ncbi .nlm.nih.gov/pubmed/19440139

17 Freedman BR, Gordon JA, Soslowsky LJ. *The Achilles tendon: fundamental properties and mechanisms governing healing.* Muscles Ligaments Tendons J. 2014 Jul 14;4(2):245-55. https://www.ncbi.nlm.nih.gov/pmc/articles/PMC4187594/

18 Pufe T, Peterson WJ, Mentlein R, Tillmann BN. *The role of vasculature and angiogenesis for the pathogenesis of degenerative tendon disease.* Scand J Med Sci Sports 2005;15(4):211–222. https://www.ncbi.nlm.nih.gov/pubmed/15998338

19 Cook JL, Khan KM, Purdam C. *Achilles tendinopathy.* Man Ther. 2002 Aug;7(3):121-30. https://www.ncbi.nlm.nih.gov /pubmed/12372309

20 Hayem G. *Tenology: a new fontier.* Joint Bone Spine 2001;68:19–25. https://www.ncbi.nlm.nih.gov/pubmed/11235776

21 Freedman BR, Gordon JA, Soslowsky LJ. *The Achilles tendon: fundamental properties and mechanisms governing healing.* Muscles Ligaments Tendons J. 2014 Jul 14;4(2):245-55. https://www.ncbi.nlm.nih.gov/pmc/articles/PMC4187594/

22 Alfredson H, Thorsen K, Lorentzon R, et al. *In situ microdialysis in tendon tissue: high levels of glutamate, but not prostaglandin E2 in chronic Achilles tendon pain.* Knee Surg Sports Traumatol Arthrosc. 1999;7(6):378-81. https://www.ncbi.nlm.nih.gov/pubmed/10639657

23 Tan SC, Chan O. *Achilles and patellar tendinopathy: current understanding of pathophysiology and management.* Disabil Rehabil. 2008;30(20-22):1608-15. https://www.ncbi.nlm.nih.gov/pubmed/19005917

24 Jarvinen M, Jozsa L, Kannus P, Jarvinen TL, Kvist M, Leadbetter W. *Histopathological findings in chronic tendon disorders.* Scan J Med Sci Sports 1997;7:86-95. https://www.ncbi.nlm.nih.gov/pubmed/9211609

25 Riley, Graham Peter. *Tendon and ligament biochemistry and pathology.* Oxford University Press. January 2011. Pg 25-28

26 Joseph MF, Denegar CR. *Treating tendinopathy: perspective on anti-inflammatory intervention and therapeutic exercise.* Send to Clin Sports Med. 2015 Apr;34(2):363-74. doi: 10.1016/j.csm.2014.12.006. Epub 2015 Jan 24. https://www.ncbi.nlm.nih.gov/pubmed/25818719

27 Kane, Justin. *Achilles Tendon Rupture.* American Orthopaedic Foot and Ankle Society. 2015 Jul. Accessed 15 1 2019. www.aofas.org/PRC/conditions/Pages/Conditions/Achilles-Tendon-Rupture.aspx

28 Jozsa L1, Kannus P. *Histopathological findings in spontaneous tendon ruptures.* Scand J Med Sci Sports. 1997 Apr;7(2):113-8. https://www.ncbi.nlm.nih.gov/pubmed/9211612

29 Morgan S, Coetzee FF. *Proposing a Patellar Tendinopathy Screening tool following a systematic review.* S Afr J Physiother. 2018 Sep 26;74(1):454. doi: 10.4102/sajp.v74i1.454. eCollection 2018. https://www.ncbi.nlm.nih.gov/pmc/articles/pmid/30349877/

30 Hodgson RJ, O'Connor PJ, Grainger AJ. *Tendon and ligament imaging.* Br J Radiol. 2012 Aug;85(1016):1157-72. doi: 10.1259/bjr/34786470. Epub 2012 May 2. https://www.ncbi.nlm.nih.gov/pmc/articles/pmid/22553301/

31 Chang A, Miller TT. *Imaging of tendons.* Sports Health. 2009 Jul;1(4):293-300. https://www.ncbi.nlm.nih.gov/pmc/articles/pmid/23015886/

32 Brinjikji W, Luetmer PH, Comstock B. *Systematic literature review of imaging features of spinal degeneration in asymptomatic populations.* AJNR Am J Neuroradiol. 2015 Apr;36(4):811-6. doi: 10.3174/ajnr.A4173. Epub 2014 Nov 27. https://www.ncbi.nlm.nih.gov/pmc/articles/pmid/25430861/

33 Kannus P, Jozsa L. *Histopathological changes preceding spontaneous rupture of a tendon.* A controlled study of 891 patients. J Bone Joint Surg Am. 1991 Dec;73(10):1507-25. https://www.ncbi.nlm.nih.gov/pubmed/1748700

34 Fredberg U, Stengaard-Pedersen K. *Chronic tendinopathy tissue pathology, pain mechanisms, and etiology with a special focus on inflammation.* Scand J Med Sci Sports. 2008 Feb;18(1):3-15. doi: 10.1111/j.1600-0838.2007.00746.x. https://onlinelibrary.wiley.com/doi/full/10.1111/j.1600-0838.2007.00746.x

35 Noback PC, Freibott CE, Tantigate D, et al. *Prevalence of Asymptomatic Achilles Tendinosis.* Foot Ankle Int. 2018 Oct;39(10):1205-1209. doi: 10.1177/1071100718778592. Epub 2018 Jun 1. https://www.ncbi.nlm.nih.gov/pubmed/29855207

36 Joseph MF, Trojian TH, Anderson JM, et al. *Incidence of morphologic changes in asymptomatic Achilles tendons in an active young adult population.* J Sport Rehabil. 2012 Aug;21(3):249-52. https://www.ncbi.nlm.nih.gov/pubmed/22894979

37 Abate M, Salini V, Antinolfi P, Schiavone C. *Ultrasound morphology of the Achilles in asymptomatic patients with and without diabetes.* Foot Ankle Int. 2014 Jan;35(1):44-9. doi: 10.1177/1071100713510496. Epub 2013 Oct 25. https://www.ncbi.nlm.nih.gov/pubmed/24163317

38 Bley B, Abid W. *Imaging of Tendinopathy: A Physician's Perspective.* J Orthop Sports Phys Ther. 2015 Nov;45(11):826-8. doi: 10.2519/jospt.2015.0113. https://www.jospt.org/doi/full/10.2519/jospt.2015.0113

39 Docking SI, Cook J. How do tendons adapt? Going beyond tissue responses to understand positive adaptation and pathology development: A narrative review. J Musculoskelet Neuronal Interact. 2019 Sep 1;19(3):300-310. https://www.ncbi.nlm.nih.gov/pmc/articles/pmid/31475937/

40 Blazina ME, Kerlan RK, Jobe FW, Carter VS, Carlson GJ. *Jumper's knee.* Orthop Clin North Am. 1973 Jul;4(3):665-78. https://www.ncbi.nlm.nih.gov/pubmed/4783891

41 *Published Guidelines.* Academy of Orthopaedic Physical Therapy. 15 1 2019. www.orthopt.org/content/practice/clinical-practice-guidelines addendum for mid-portion Achilles: https://www.jospt.org/doi/pdfplus/10.2519/jospt.2018.0302

42 J Robinson, J Cook, C Purdam, P Visentini, J Ross, N Maffulli, J Taunton, and K Khan. *The VISA-A questionnaire: a valid and reliable index of the clinical severity of Achilles tendinopathy.* Br J Sports Med. 2001 Oct; 35(5): 335–341. https://www.ncbi.nlm.nih.gov/pmc/articles/PMC1724384/

43   Reb CW, Saini SS, Stenson JF, Albana MF, Pedowitz DI, Raikin SM, Daniel JN. Content Relevance of the Foot and Ankle Ability Measure in Patients With Achilles Tendon Diseases. Foot Ankle Spec. 2018 Jun;11(3):217-222. doi: 10.1177/1938640017718342. Epub 2017 Jul 12. https://www.ncbi.nlm.nih.gov/pubmed/28699355

44   McCormack J, Underwood F, Slaven E, Cappaert T. *THE MINIMUM CLINICALLY IMPORTANT DIFFERENCE ON THE VISA-A AND LEFS FOR PATIENTS WITH INSERTIONAL ACHILLES TENDINOPATHY.* Int J Sports Phys Ther. 2015 Oct; 10(5): 639–644. https://www.ncbi.nlm.nih.gov/pmc/articles/PMC4595917/

45   Roberts LA, Raastad T, Markworth JF, Figueiredo VC. *Post-exercise cold water immersion attenuates acute anabolic signalling and long-term adaptations in muscle to strength training.* J Physiol. 2015 Sep 15;593(18):4285-301. doi: 10.1113/JP270570. Epub 2015 Aug 13. https://www.ncbi.nlm.nih.gov/pmc/articles/pmid/26174323/

46   Broatch JR, Petersen A, Bishop DJ. *The Influence of Post-Exercise Cold-Water Immersion on Adaptive Responses to Exercise: A Review of the Literature.* Sports Med. 2018 Jun;48(6):1369-1387. doi: 10.1007/s40279-018-0910-8. https://www.ncbi.nlm.nih.gov/pubmed/29627884

47   Trappe TA, White F, Lambert CP, Cesar D. *Effect of ibuprofen and acetaminophen on postexercise muscle protein synthesis.* Am J Physiol Endocrinol Metab. 2002 Mar;282(3):E551-6. https://www.ncbi.nlm.nih.gov/pubmed/11832356

48   Lundberg TR, Howatson G. *Analgesic and anti-inflammatory drugs in sports: Implications for exercise performance and training adaptations.* Scand J Med Sci Sports. 2018 Nov;28(11):2252-2262. doi: 10.1111/sms.13275. Epub 2018 Sep 2. https://www.ncbi.nlm.nih.gov/pubmed/30102811

49   McAuliffe S, McCreesh K, Culloty F. *Can ultrasound imaging predict the development of Achilles and patellar tendinopathy? A systematic review and meta-analysis.* Br J Sports Med. 2016 Dec;50(24):1516-1523. doi: 10.1136/bjsports-2016-096288. Epub 2016 Sep 15. https://www.ncbi.nlm.nih.gov/pubmed/27633025

50   Lewis JS, Sandford FM. *Rotator cuff tendinopathy: is there a role for polyunsaturated Fatty acids and antioxidants?* J Hand Ther. 2009 Jan-Mar;22(1):49-55; quiz 56. doi: 10.1197/j.jht.2008.06.007. Epub 2008 Aug 30. https://www.ncbi.nlm.nih.gov/pubmed/18950988

51   De Marchi A, Pozza S, Cenna E. *In Achilles tendinopathy, the neovascularization, detected by contrast-enhanced ultrasound (CEUS), is abundant but not related to symptoms.* Knee Surg Sports Traumatol Arthrosc. 2018 Jul;26(7):2051-2058. doi: 10.1007/s00167-017-4710-8. Epub 2017 Oct 27. https://www.ncbi.nlm.nih.gov/pubmed/29079961

52   Li HY, Hua YH. Achilles Tendinopathy: *Current Concepts about the Basic Science and Clinical Treatments.* Biomed Res Int. 2016;2016:6492597. Epub 2016 Nov 3. https://www.ncbi.nlm.nih.gov/pmc/articles/pmid/27885357/

53   Garra G1, Singer AJ, Leno R. *Heat or cold packs for neck and back strain: a randomized controlled trial of efficacy.* Acad Emerg Med. 2010 May;17(5):484-9. doi: 10.1111/j.1553-2712.2010.00735.x. https://www.ncbi.nlm.nih.gov/pubmed/20536800

54   Magnusson SP, Langberg H, Kjaer M. *The pathogenesis of tendinopathy: Balancing the response to loading.* Nature Reviews Rheumatology 2010 March:6(5):262-8. https://www.researchgate.net/publication/42389969_The_pathogenesis_of_tendinopathy_Balancing_the_response_to_loading

55   Alfredson H, Pietilä T, Jonsson P, Lorentzon R, et al. *Heavy-load eccentric calf muscle training for the treatment of chronic Achilles tendinosis.* Am J Sports Med. 1998 May-Jun;26(3):360-6. https://www.ncbi.nlm.nih.gov/pubmed/9617396

56   Stanish WD, Rubinovich RM, Curwin S. *Eccentric exercise in chronic tendonitis.* Clin Orthop Relat Res. 1986 Jul;(208):65-8. https://www.ncbi.nlm.nih.gov/pubmed/3720143

57   Silbernagel KG, Thomee R, Thomee P, Karlsson J, et al. *Eccentric overload training for patients with chronic Achilles tendon pain--a randomised controlled study with reliability testing of the evaluation methods.* Scand J Med Sci Sports. 2001 Aug;11(4):197-206. https://www.ncbi.nlm.nih.gov/pubmed/11476424

58   Drew BT, Smith TO, Littlewood C, Sturrock B. *Do structural changes (eg, collagen/matrix) explain the response to therapeutic exercises in tendinopathy: a systematic review.* Br J Sports Med. 2014 Jun;48(12):966-72. doi: 10.1136/bjsports-2012-091285. Epub 2012 Oct 31. https://www.ncbi.nlm.nih.gov/pubmed/23118117

59   Couppe C, Svensson RB, Silbernagel KG, Langberg H, Magnusson SP. *Eccentric or Concentric Exercises for the Treatment of Tendinopathies?* J Orthop Sports Phys Ther. 2015 Nov;45(11):853-63. doi: 10.2519/jospt.2015.5910. Epub 2015 Oct 15. https://www.researchgate.net/publication/282911158_Eccentric_or_Concentric_Exercises_for_the_Treatment_of_Tendinopathies

60   Stasinopoulos D, Stasinopoulos I. *Comparison of effects of eccentric training, eccentric-concentric training, and eccentric-concentric training combined with isometric contraction in the treatment of lateral elbow tendinopathy.* J Hand Ther. 2017 Jan - Mar;30(1):13-19. doi: 10.1016/j.jht.2016.09.001. Epub 2016 Nov 4. https://www.sciencedirect.com/science/article/pii/S0894113016301302

61 Bohm S, Mersmann F, Arampatzis A. Human tendon adaptation in response to mechanical loading: a systematic review and meta-analysis of exercise intervention studies on healthy adults. Sports Med Open. 2015 Dec;1(1):7. Epub 2015 Mar 27. https://www.ncbi.nlm.nih.gov/pmc/articles/PMC4532714/

62 Kubo K, Kanehisa H, Fukunaga T. *Effects of different duration isometric contractions on tendon elasticity in human quadriceps muscles.* J Physiol. 2001 Oct 15;536(Pt 2):649-55. https://www.ncbi.nlm.nih.gov/pmc/articles/PMC2278867/

63 Malliaras P, Barton CJ, Reeves ND, Langberg H, et al. *Achilles and patellar tendinopathy loading programmes: a systematic review comparing clinical outcomes and identifying potential mechanisms for effectiveness.* Sports Med. 2013 Apr;43(4):267-86. doi: 10.1007/s40279-013-0019-z. https://www.ncbi.nlm.nih.gov/pubmed/23494258

64 *Achilles Tendinopathy Toolkit: Appendix A.* Physiopedia. 05 3 2019. https://www.physio-pedia.com/Achilles_Tendinopathy_Toolkit:_Appendix_A

65 Schoenfeld BJ, Ogborn D, Krieger JW. *Effects of Resistance Training Frequency on Measures of Muscle Hypertrophy: A Systematic Review and Meta-Analysis.* Sports Med. 2016 Nov;46(11):1689-1697. doi: 10.1007/s40279-016-0543-8. https://www.ncbi.nlm.nih.gov/pubmed/27102172

66 Dankel SJ, Mattocks KT, Jessee MB, Buckner SL. *Frequency: The Overlooked Resistance Training Variable for Inducing Muscle Hypertrophy?* Sports Med. 2017 May;47(5):799-805. doi: 10.1007/s40279-016-0640-8. https://www.ncbi.nlm.nih.gov/pubmed/27752983

67 McMaster DT, Gill N, Cronin J, McGuigan M. *The development, retention and decay rates of strength and power in elite rugby union, rugby league and American football: a systematic review.* Sports Med. 2013 May;43(5):367-84. doi: 10.1007/s40279-013-0031-3.

68 Tzur A, Roberts B. *Scientific Recommendations for Strength and Hypertrophy Training from 150+ Studies (part 1 of 3).* The Science of Fitness - SCI-FIT. 2017 04 03. Scihttps://sci-fit.net/scientific-recommendations-1/

69 Nuckols G. *The "Hypertrophy Rep Range" – Fact or Fiction?* Stronger by Science. 2016 Feb 25. https://www.strongerbyscience.com/hypertrophy-range-fact-fiction/

70 American College of Sports Medicine. *American College of Sports Medicine position stand. Progression models in resistance training for healthy adults.* Med Sci Sports Exerc. 2009 Mar;41(3):687-708. doi: 10.1249/MSS.0b013e3181915670. https://www.ncbi.nlm.nih.gov/pubmed/19204579

71 Stasinopoulos D, Malliaras P. *Is the heavy slow resistance program effective for all patients with tendinopathy and effective for all its sites?* J Sports Med Phys Fitness. 2016 Nov;56(11):1430-1431. https://www.researchgate.net/publication/311299294_Is_the_heavy_slow_resistance_program_effective_for_all_patients_with_tendinopathy_and_effective_for_all_its_sites

72 Beyer R, Kongsgaard M, Hougs Kjaer B. *Heavy Slow Resistance Versus Eccentric Training as Treatment for Achilles Tendinopathy: A Randomized Controlled Trial.* Am J Sports Med. 2015 Jul;43(7):1704-11. doi: 10.1177/0363546515584760. Epub 2015 May 27. https://www.ncbi.nlm.nih.gov/pubmed/26018970

73 Lim HY, Wong SH. *Effects of isometric, eccentric, or heavy slow resistance exercises on pain and function in individuals with patellar tendinopathy: A systematic review.* Physiother Res Int. 2018 Oct;23(4):e1721. doi: 10.1002/pri.1721. Epub 2018 Jul 4. https://www.ncbi.nlm.nih.gov/pubmed/29972281

74 Brox JI, Storheim K, Grotle M, Tveito TH, Indahl A, Eriksen HR. *Systematic review of back schools, brief education, and fear-avoidance training for chronic low back pain.* Spine J. 2008 Nov-Dec;8(6):948-58. Epub 2007 Nov 19. https://www.ncbi.nlm.nih.gov/pubmed/18024224

75 Melzack R. *Pain and the neuromatrix in the brain.* J Dent Educ. 2001 Dec;65(12):1378-82. https://www.ncbi.nlm.nih.gov/pubmed/11780656

76 Gatchel RJ, Peng YB, Peters ML, Fuchs PN, Turk DC. *The biopsychosocial approach to chronic pain: scientific advances and future directions.* Psychol Bull. 2007 Jul;133(4):581-624. https://www.ncbi.nlm.nih.gov/pubmed/17592957

77 Butler, David & Moseley, Lorimer. *Explain pain 2nd Edition.* Noigroup Publications, Sept 2013. Print.

78 Louw A, Diener I, Butler DS, Puentedura EJ. *The effect of neuroscience education on pain, disability, anxiety, and stress in chronic musculoskeletal pain.* Arch Phys Med Rehabil. 2011 Dec;92(12):2041-56. doi: 10.1016/j.apmr.2011.07.198. https://www.ncbi.nlm.nih.gov/pubmed/22133255

79 Ryan CG, Gray HG, Newton M, Granat MH. *Pain biology education and exercise classes compared to pain biology education alone for individuals with chronic low back pain: a pilot randomised controlled trial.* Man Ther. 2010 Aug;15(4):382-7. doi: 10.1016/j.math.2010.03.003. Epub 2010 Mar 31. https://www.ncbi.nlm.nih.gov/pubmed/20359937

80 Moseley GL, Nicholas MK, Hodges PW. *A randomized controlled trial of intensive neurophysiology education in chronic low back pain.* Clin J Pain. 2004 Sep-Oct;20(5):324-30. https://www.ncbi.nlm.nih.gov/pubmed/15322439

81 Koes BW, van Tulder M, Lin CW, et al. *An updated overview of clinical guidelines for the management of non-specific low back pain in primary care.* Eur Spine J. 2010 Dec;19(12):2075-94. doi: 10.1007/s00586-010-1502-y. Epub 2010 Jul 3. https://www.ncbi.nlm.nih.gov/pmc/articles/pmid/20602122/

82 Traeger AC, Moseley GL, Hubscher M, et al. *Pain education to prevent chronic low back pain: a study protocol for a randomised controlled trial.* BMJ Open. 2014 Jun 2;4(6):e005505. doi: 10.1136/bmjopen-2014-005505. https://www.ncbi.nlm.nih.gov/pmc/articles/PMC4054624/

83 Moseley GL, Gallace A, Spence C. *Bodily illusions in health and disease: physiological and clinical perspectives and the concept of a cortical 'body matrix'.* Neurosci Biobehav Rev. 2012 Jan;36(1):34-46. doi: 10.1016/j.neubiorev.2011.03.013. Epub 2011 Apr 6. https://www.ncbi.nlm.nih.gov/pubmed/21477616

84 Louw A, Zimney K, Puentedura EJ, Diener I. The efficacy of pain neuroscience education on musculoskeletal pain: A systematic review of the literature. Physiother Theory Pract. 2016 Jul;32(5):332-55. doi: 10.1080/09593985.2016.1194646. Epub 2016 Jun 28. http://accurateclinic.com/wp-content/uploads/2016/03/The-clinical-application-of-teaching-people-about-pain-2016.pdf

85 Puentedura EJ, Flynn T. *Combining manual therapy with pain neuroscience education in the treatment of chronic low back pain: A narrative review of the literature.* Physiother Theory Pract. 2016 Jul;32(5):408-14. doi: 10.1080/09593985.2016.1194663. Epub 2016 Jun 30. https://www.ncbi.nlm.nih.gov/pubmed/27362980

86 Blickenstaff C, Pearson N. *Reconciling movement and exercise with pain neuroscience education: A case for consistent education.* Physiother Theory Pract. 2016 Jul;32(5):396-407. doi: 10.1080/09593985.2016.1194653. Epub 2016 Jun 29. https://www.ncbi.nlm.nih.gov/pubmed/27356079

87 Louw A, Zimney K, O'Hotto C, Hilton S. *The clinical application of teaching people about pain.* Physiother Theory Pract. 2016 Jul;32(5):385-95. doi: 10.1080/09593985.2016.1194652. Epub 2016 Jun 28. https://www.ncbi.nlm.nih.gov/pubmed/27351903

88 Rio E, Moseley L, Purdam C, Samiric T. *The pain of tendinopathy: physiological or pathophysiological?* Sports Med. 2014 Jan;44(1):9-23. doi: 10.1007/s40279-013-0096-z. https://www.ncbi.nlm.nih.gov/pubmed/24027089

89 Raney EB, Thankam FG, Dilisio MF, Agrawal DK. *Pain and the pathogenesis of biceps tendinopathy.* Am J Transl Res. 2017 Jun 15;9(6):2668-2683. eCollection 2017. https://www.ncbi.nlm.nih.gov/pmc/articles/PMC5489872/

90 Mascaro A, Cos MA, Morral A, Roig A, Purdam C, Cook J. *Load management in tendinopathy: Clinical progression for Achilles and patellar tendinopathy.* Apunts. Medicina de l'Esport 2018 Jan–Mar:53(197):19-27

91 Rio E, Kidgell D, Purdam C, Gaida J, Moseley GL, Pearce AJ, Cook, J. *Isometric exercise induces analgesia and reduces inhibition in patellar tendinopathy.* Br J Sports Med. 2015 Oct;49(19):1277-83. doi: 10.1136/bjsports-2014-094386. Epub 2015 May 15. https://bjsm.bmj.com/content/49/19/1277.long

92 Rio E, van Ark M, Docking S, Moseley GL, Kidgell D, Gaida JE, van den Akker-Scheek I, Zwerver J, Cook J. *Isometric Contractions Are More Analgesic Than Isotonic Contractions for Patellar Tendon Pain: An In-Season Randomized Clinical Trial.* Clin J Sport Med. 2017 May;27(3):253-259. doi: 10.1097/JSM.0000000000000364. https://journals.lww.com/cjsportsmed/fulltext/2017/05000/Isometric_Contractions_Are_More_Analgesic_Than.3.aspx

93 van Ark M, Cook JL, Docking SI, Zwerver J, Gaida JE, van den Akker-Scheek I, Rio E. *Do isometric and isotonic exercise programs reduce pain in athletes with patellar tendinopathy in-season? A randomised clinical trial.* J Sci Med Sport. 2016 Sep;19(9):702-6. doi: 10.1016/j.jsams.2015.11.006. Epub 2015 Dec 7. https://www.ncbi.nlm.nih.gov/pubmed/26707957

94 Rio E, Purdam C, Girdwood M, Cook J. *Isometric Exercise to Reduce Pain in Patellar Tendinopathy In-Season; Is It Effective "on the Road?"* Clin J Sport Med. 2017 Nov 16. doi: 10.1097/JSM.0000000000000549. https://www.ncbi.nlm.nih.gov/pubmed/29210775

95 Pearson SJ, Stadler S, Menz H, Morrissey D, Scott I, Munteanu S, Malliaras P. *Immediate and Short-Term Effects of Short- and Long-Duration Isometric Contractions in Patellar Tendinopathy.* Clin J Sport Med. 2018 Aug 8. doi: 10.1097/JSM.0000000000000625. https://www.ncbi.nlm.nih.gov/pubmed/30095504

96 Lim HY, Wong SH. *Effects of isometric, eccentric, or heavy slow resistance exercises on pain and function in individuals with patellar tendinopathy: A systematic review.* Physiother Res Int. 2018 Oct;23(4):e1721. doi: 10.1002/pri.1721. Epub 2018 Jul 4. https://www.ncbi.nlm.nih.gov/pubmed/29972281

97 *Training Load Chart.* NSCA. 05 3 2019. https://www.nsca.com/contentassets/61d813865e264c6e852cadfe247eae52/nsca_training_load_chart.pdf

98 Low, Steven. *Overcoming Gravity: a Systematic Approach to Gymnastics and Bodyweight Strength (Second Edition).* Battle Ground Creative, 2016.

99   Exrx.net. *Predicting One-rep Max*. 2019. [online] Available at: https://exrx.net/Calculators/OneRepMax [Accessed 25 May 2019].

100   Visnes H, Bahr R. *The evolution of eccentric training as treatment for patellar tendinopathy (jumper's knee): a critical review of exercise programmes*. Br J Sports Med. 2007 Apr;41(4):217-23. Epub 2007 Jan 29. https://www.ncbi.nlm.nih.gov/pmc/articles /pmid/17261559/

101   Habets B, van Cingel RE. *Eccentric exercise training in chronic mid-portion Achilles tendinopathy: a systematic review on different protocols*. Scand J Med Sci Sports. 2015 Feb;25(1):3-15. doi: 10.1111/sms.12208. Epub 2014 Mar 20. https://www.ncbi .nlm.nih.gov/pubmed/24650048

102   Malliaras P, Barton CJ, Reeves ND, Langberg H, et al. *Achilles and patellar tendinopathy loading programmes: a systematic review comparing clinical outcomes and identifying potential mechanisms for effectiveness*. Sports Med. 2013 Apr;43(4):267-86. doi: 10.1007/s40279-013-0019-z. https://www.ncbi.nlm.nih.gov/pubmed/23494258

103   Bohm S, Mersmann F, Tettke M, et al. *Human Achilles tendon plasticity in response to cyclic strain: effect of rate and duration*. J Exp Biol. 2014 Nov 15;217(Pt 22):4010-7. doi: 10.1242/jeb.112268. Epub 2014 Sep 29. http://jeb.biologists.org/content /217/22/4010.long

104   Malliaras P, Cook J, Purdam C, Rio E, et al. *Patellar Tendinopathy: Clinical Diagnosis, Load Management, and Advice for Challenging Case Presentations*. The Journal of orthopaedic and sports physical therapy. 2015 Sep:1-33.

105   Mascaro A, Cos MA, Morral A, Roig A, Purdam C, Cook J. *Load management in tendinopathy: Clinical progression for Achilles and patellar tendinopathy*. Apunts. Medicina de l'Esport 2018 Jan–Mar:53(197):19-27 https://www.sciencedirect.com /science/article/pii/S1886658117300580#bib0430

106   Gabbett TJ. *The training-injury prevention paradox: should athletes be training smarter and harder?* Br J Sports Med. 2016 Mar;50(5):273-80. doi: 10.1136/bjsports-2015-095788. Epub 2016 Jan 12. https://bjsm.bmj.com/content/50/5/273

107   Hulin BT, Gabbett TJ, Caputi P, et al. *Low chronic workload and the acute:chronic workload ratio are more predictive of injury than between-match recovery time: a two-season prospective cohort study in elite rugby league players*. Br J Sports Med. 2016 Aug;50(16):1008-12. doi: 10.1136/bjsports-2015-095364. Epub 2016 Feb 5. https://www.ncbi.nlm.nih.gov/ pubmed/26851288

108   Hulin BT, Gabbett TJ, Lawson DW, et al. *The acute:chronic workload ratio predicts injury: high chronic workload may decrease injury risk in elite rugby league players*. Br J Sports Med. 2016 Feb;50(4):231-6. doi: 10.1136/bjsports-2015-094817. Epub 2015 Oct 28. https://www.ncbi.nlm.nih.gov/pubmed/26511006

109   Murray NB, Gabbett TJ, Townshend AD, Blanch P3. *Calculating acute:chronic workload ratios using exponentially weighted moving averages provides a more sensitive indicator of injury likelihood than rolling averages*. Br J Sports Med. 2017 May;51(9):749-754. doi: 10.1136/bjsports-2016-097152. Epub 2016 Dec 21. https://www.ncbi.nlm.nih.gov/ pubmed/28003238

110   Bowen L, Gross AS, Gimpel M, Li FX. *Accumulated workloads and the acute:chronic workload ratio relate to injury risk in elite youth football players*. Br J Sports Med. 2017 Mar;51(5):452-459. doi: 10.1136/bjsports-2015-095820. Epub 2016 Jul 22. https://www.ncbi.nlm.nih.gov/pmc/articles/pmid/27450360/

111   Bowen L, Gross AS, Gimpel M, et al. *Spikes in acute:chronic workload ratio (ACWR) associated with a 5-7 times greater injury rate in English Premier League football players: a comprehensive 3-year study*. Br J Sports Med. 2019 Feb 21. pii: bjsports-2018-099422. doi: 10.1136/bjsports-2018-099422. [Epub ahead of print]. https://www.ncbi.nlm.nih.gov/ pubmed/30792258

112   Weiss KJ, Allen SV, McGuigan MR, Whatman CS. *The Relationship Between Training Load and Injury in Men's Professional Basketball*. Int J Sports Physiol Perform. 2017 Oct;12(9):1238-1242. doi: 10.1123/ijspp.2016-0726. Epub 2017 Mar 2. https://www.ncbi.nlm.nih.gov/pubmed/28253031

113   Sampson JA, Murray A, Williams S, et al. *Injury risk-workload associations in NCAA American college football*. J Sci Med Sport. 2018 Dec;21(12):1215-1220. doi: 10.1016/j.jsams.2018.05.019. Epub 2018 May 22. https://www.ncbi.nlm.nih.gov /pubmed/29843960

114   Malone S, Owen A, Newton M, et al. *The acute:chronic workload ratio in relation to injury risk in professional soccer*. J Sci Med Sport. 2017 Jun;20(6):561-565. doi: 10.1016/j.jsams.2016.10.014. Epub 2016 Nov 9. https://www.ncbi.nlm.nih.gov/ pubmed/27856198

115   Kim HG, Cheon EJ, Bai DS, et al. *Stress and Heart Rate Variability: A Meta-Analysis and Review of the Literature*. Psychiatry Investig. 2018 Mar;15(3):235-245. doi: 10.30773/pi.2017.08.17. Epub 2018 Feb 28. https://www.ncbi.nlm.nih.gov/pmc/ articles/pmid/29486547/

116 Sekiguchi Y, Huggins RA, Curtis RM, et al. *Relationship Between Heart Rate Variability and Acute: Chronic Load Ratio Throughout a Season in NCAA D1 Men's Soccer Players.* J Strength Cond Res. 2018 Oct 4. doi: 10.1519/JSC.0000000000002853. [Epub ahead of print] https://www.ncbi.nlm.nih.gov/pubmed/30289866

117 Williams S, Booton T, Watson M, et al. *Heart Rate Variability is a Moderating Factor in the Workload-Injury Relationship of Competitive CrossFit™ Athletes.* J Sports Sci Med. 2017 Dec 1;16(4):443-449. eCollection 2017 Dec. https://www.ncbi.nlm.nih.gov/pmc/articles/pmid/29238242/

118 Baumert M, Brechtel L, Lock J, et al. *Heart rate variability, blood pressure variability, and baroreflex sensitivity in overtrained athletes.* Clin J Sport Med. 2006 Sep;16(5):412-7. https://www.ncbi.nlm.nih.gov/pubmed/17016118

119 Rusciano A, Corradini G, Stoianov I. *Neuroplus biofeedback improves attention, resilience, and injury prevention in elite soccer players.* Psychophysiology. 2017 Jun;54(6):916-926. doi: 10.1111/psyp.12847. Epub 2017 Feb 21. https://www.ncbi.nlm.nih.gov/pubmed/28220500

120 Hellard P, Guimaraes F, Avalos M, et al. *Modeling the association between HR variability and illness in elite swimmers.* Med Sci Sports Exerc. 2011 Jun;43(6):1063-70. doi: 10.1249/MSS.0b013e318204de1c. https://www.ncbi.nlm.nih.gov/pmc/articles/pmid/21085039/

CHAPTER 8 BIBLIOGRAPHY

Eccentric References

Tan SC, Chan O. *Achilles and patellar tendinopathy: current understanding of pathophysiology and management.* Disabil Rehabil. 2008;30(20-22): 1608-15. doi: 10.1080/09638280701792268. https://www.ncbi.nlm.nih.gov/pubmed/19005917

Al-Abbad H, Simon JV. *The effectiveness of extracorporeal shock wave therapy on chronic achilles tendinopathy: a systematic review.* Foot Ankle Int. 2013 Jan;34(1):33-41. doi: 10.1177/1071100712464354. https://www.ncbi.nlm.nih.gov/pubmed/23386759

Kingma JJ, de Knikker R, Wittink HM, Takken T. *Eccentric overload training in patients with chronic Achilles tendinopathy: a systematic review.* Br J Sports Med. 2007 Jun;41(6):e3. Epub 2006 Oct 11. https://www.ncbi.nlm.nih.gov/pmc/articles/PMC2465314/

Kearney R, Costa ML. *Insertional achilles tendinopathy management: a systematic review.* Foot Ankle Int. 2010 Aug;31(8):689-94. doi: 10.3113/FAI.2010.0689. https://www.ncbi.nlm.nih.gov/pubmed/20727317

Wiegerinck JI, Kerkhoffs GM, van Sterkenburg MN, Sierevelt IN, van Dijk CN. *Treatment for insertional Achilles tendinopathy: a systematic review.* Knee Surg Sports Traumatol Arthrosc. 2013 Jun;21(6):1345-55. doi: 10.1007/s00167-012-2219-8. Epub 2012 Oct 6. https://www.ncbi.nlm.nih.gov/pubmed/23052113

Woitzik E, Jacobs C, Wong JJ, Côté P, et al. *The effectiveness of exercise on recovery and clinical outcomes of soft tissue injuries of the leg, ankle, and foot: A systematic review by the Ontario Protocol for Traffic Injury Management (OPTIMa) Collaboration.* Man Ther. 2015 Oct;20(5):633-45. doi: 10.1016/j.math.2015.03.012. Epub 2015 Mar 28. https://www.ncbi.nlm.nih.gov/pubmed/25892707

Sussmilch-Leitch SP, Collins NJ, Bialocerkowski AE, Warden SJ, Crossley KM. *Physical therapies for Achilles tendinopathy: systematic review and meta-analysis.* J Foot Ankle Res. 2012 Jul 2;5(1):15. doi: 10.1186/1757-1146-5-15. https://www.ncbi.nlm.nih.gov/pmc/articles/PMC3537637/

Magnussen RA, Dunn WR, Thomson AB. *Nonoperative treatment of midportion Achilles tendinopathy: a systematic review.* Clin J Sport Med. 2009 Jan;19(1):54-64. doi: 10.1097/JSM.0b013e31818ef090. https://www.ncbi.nlm.nih.gov/pubmed/19124985

Wasielewski NJ, Kotsko KM. *Does eccentric exercise reduce pain and improve strength in physically active adults with symptomatic lower extremity tendinosis? A systematic review.* J Athl Train. 2007 Jul-Sep;42(3):409-21. https://www.ncbi.nlm.nih.gov/pmc/articles/PMC1978463/

Habets B, van Cingel RE. *Eccentric exercise training in chronic mid-portion Achilles tendinopathy: a systematic review on different protocols.* Scand J Med Sci Sports. 2015 Feb;25(1):3-15. doi: 10.1111/sms.12208. Epub 2014 Mar 20. https://www.ncbi.nlm.nih.gov/pubmed/24650048

Woodley BL, Newsham-West RJ, Baxter GD. *Chronic tendinopathy: effectiveness of eccentric exercise.* Br J Sports Med. 2007 Apr;41(4):188-98; discussion 199. Epub 2006 Oct 24. https://www.ncbi.nlm.nih.gov/pmc/articles/PMC2658941/

Frizziero A, Trainito S, Oliva F, Nicoli Aldini N, Masiero S, Maffulli N. *The role of eccentric exercise in sport injuries rehabilitation.* Br Med Bull. 2014 Jun;110(1):47-75. doi: 10.1093/bmb/ldu006. Epub 2014 Apr 15. https://www.ncbi.nlm.nih.gov/pubmed/24736013

Malliaras P, Barton CJ, Reeves ND, Langberg H. *Achilles and patellar tendinopathy loading programmes: a systematic review comparing clinical outcomes and identifying potential mechanisms for effectiveness.* Sports Med. 2013 Apr;43(4):267-86. doi: 10.1007/s40279-013-0019-z. https://www.ncbi.nlm.nih.gov/pubmed/23494258

Andres BM, Murrell GA. *Treatment of tendinopathy: what works, what does not, and what is on the horizon.* Clin Orthop Relat Res. 2008 Jul;466(7):1539-54. doi: 10.1007/s11999-008-0260-1. Epub 2008 Apr 30. https://www.ncbi.nlm.nih.gov/pmc/articles/PMC2505250/

Larsson ME, Käll I, Nilsson-Helander K. *Treatment of patellar tendinopathy--a systematic review of randomized controlled trials.* Knee Surg Sports Traumatol Arthrosc. 2012 Aug;20(8):1632-46. doi: 10.1007/s00167-011-1825-1. Epub 2011 Dec 21. https://www.ncbi.nlm.nih.gov/pubmed/22186923

Saithna A, Gogna R, Baraza N, Modi C, Spencer S. *Eccentric Exercise Protocols for Patella Tendinopathy: Should we Really be Withdrawing Athletes from Sport?* Open Orthop J. 2012;6:553-7. doi: 10.2174/1874325001206010553. Epub 2012 Nov 30. https://www.ncbi.nlm.nih.gov/pmc/articles/PMC3522085/

Malliaras P, Maffulli N, Garau G. *Eccentric training programmes in the management of lateral elbow tendinopathy.* Disabil Rehabil. 2008;30(20-22):1590-6. doi: 10.1080/09638280701786195. https://www.ncbi.nlm.nih.gov/pubmed/18608381

Johnson GW, Cadwallader K, Scheffel SB, Epperly TD. *Treatment of lateral epicondylitis.* Am Fam Physician. 2007 Sep 15;76(6):843-8. https://www.aafp.org/afp/2007/0915/p843.html

Cullinane FL, Boocock MG, Trevelyan FC. *Is eccentric exercise an effective treatment for lateral epicondylitis? A systematic review.* Clin Rehabil. 2014 Jan;28(1):3-19. doi: 10.1177/0269215513491974. Epub 2013 Jul 23. https://www.ncbi.nlm.nih.gov/pubmed/23881334

Hoogvliet P, Randsdorp MS, Dingemanse R, Koes BW, Huisstede BM. *Does effectiveness of exercise therapy and mobilisation techniques offer guidance for the treatment of lateral and medial epicondylitis? A systematic review.* Br J Sports Med. 2013 Nov;47(17):1112-9. doi: 10.1136/bjsports-2012-091990. Epub 2013 May 24. https://bjsm.bmj.com/content/47/17/1112.long

Olaussen M, Holmedal O, Lindbaek M, et al. *Treating lateral epicondylitis with corticosteroid injections or non-electrotherapeutical physiotherapy: a systematic review.* BMJ Open 2013;3:e003564. doi: 10.1136/bmjopen-2013-003564. https://bmjopen.bmj.com/content/3/10/e003564

Long L, Briscoe S, Cooper C, Hyde C, Crathorne L. *What is the clinical effectiveness and cost-effectiveness of conservative interventions for tendinopathy? An overview of systematic reviews of clinical effectiveness and systematic review of economic evaluations.* Health Technol Assess. 2015 Jan;19(8):1-134. doi: 10.3310/hta19080. https://www.ncbi.nlm.nih.gov/books/NBK269589/

Menta R, Randhawa K, Cote P, Wong JJ, et al. *The effectiveness of exercise for the management of musculoskeletal disorders and injuries of the elbow, forearm, wrist, and hand: a systematic review by the Ontario Protocol for Traffic Injury Management (OPTIMa) collaboration.* J Manipulative Physiol Ther. 2015 Sep;38(7):507-20. doi: 10.1016/j.jmpt.2015.06.002. Epub 2015 Jun 27. https://www.jmptonline.org/article/S0161-4754(15)00064-0/fulltext

Sutton D, Gross DP, Cote P, Randhawa K, et al. *Multimodal care for the management of musculoskeletal disorders of the elbow, forearm, wrist and hand: a systematic review by the Ontario Protocol for Traffic Injury Management (OPTIMa) Collaboration.* Chiropr Man Therap. 2016 Mar 7;24:8. doi: 10.1186/s12998-016-0089-8. eCollection 2016. https://www.ncbi.nlm.nih.gov/pmc/articles/PMC4780149/

Gaujoux-Viala C, Dougados M, Gossec L. *Efficacy and safety of steroid injections for shoulder and elbow tendonitis: a meta-analysis of randomised controlled trials.* Ann Rheum Dis. 2009 Dec;68(12):1843-9. doi: 10.1136/ard.2008.099572. Epub 2008 Dec 3. https://www.ncbi.nlm.nih.gov/pmc/articles/PMC2770107/

Camargo PR, Alburquerque-Sendín F, Salvini TF. *Eccentric training as a new approach for rotator cuff tendinopathy: Review and perspectives.* World J Orthop. 2014 Nov 18;5(5):634-44. doi: 10.5312/wjo.v5.i5.634. eCollection 2014 Nov 18. https://www.ncbi.nlm.nih.gov/pmc/articles/PMC4133471/

Greis AC, Derrington SM, McAuliffe M. *Evaluation and nonsurgical management of rotator cuff calcific tendinopathy.* Orthop Clin North Am. 2015 Apr;46(2):293-302. doi: 10.1016/j.ocl.2014.11.011. Epub 2015 Jan 27. https://www.ncbi.nlm.nih.gov/pubmed/25771323

Lempainen L, Johansson K, Banke IJ, Ranne J, et al. *Expert opinion: diagnosis and treatment of proximal hamstring tendinopathy.* Muscles Ligaments Tendons J. 2015 Mar 27;5(1):23-8. eCollection 2015 Jan-Mar. https://www.ncbi.nlm.nih.gov/pmc/articles/PMC4396672/

Rowe V, Hemmings S, Barton C, et al. *Conservative management of midportion Achilles tendinopathy: a mixed methods study, integrating systematic review and clinical reasoning.* Sports Med. 2012 Nov 1;42(11):941-67. doi: 10.2165/11635410-000000000-00000. https://www.ncbi.nlm.nih.gov/pubmed/23006143

Färnqvist K, Malliaras P, Pearson S. *Eccentric Exercise, Tendon Thickness, Pain and Function in Achilles Tendinopathy: A Systematic Review.* J Sport Rehabil. 2019 Mar 12:1-30. doi: 10.1123/jsr.2018-0353. [Epub ahead of print]. https://www.ncbi.nlm.nih.gov/pubmed/30860421

Ross MH, Smith MD, Mellor R, Vicenzino B. *Exercise for posterior tibial tendon dysfunction: a systematic review of randomised clinical trials and clinical guidelines.* BMJ Open Sport Exerc Med. 2018 Sep 19;4(1):e000430. doi: 10.1136/bmjsem-2018-000430. eCollection 2018. https://www.ncbi.nlm.nih.gov/pmc/articles/pmid/30271611/

Wilson F, Walshe M, O'Dwyer T, et al. *Exercise, orthoses and splinting for treating Achilles tendinopathy: a systematic review with meta-analysis.* Br J Sports Med. 2018 Dec;52(24):1564-1574. doi: 10.1136/bjsports-2017-098913. Epub 2018 Aug 31. https://www.ncbi.nlm.nih.gov/pubmed/30170996

Lucado AM, Dale RB, Vincent J, Day JM. *Do joint mobilizations assist in the recovery of lateral elbow tendinopathy? A systematic review and meta-analysis.* J Hand Ther. 2019 Apr - Jun;32(2):262-276.e1. doi: 10.1016/j.jht.2018.01.010. Epub 2018 Apr 26. https://www.ncbi.nlm.nih.gov/pubmed/29705077

Everhart JS, Cole D, Sojka JH, et al. *Treatment Options for Patellar Tendinopathy: A Systematic Review.* Arthroscopy. 2017 Apr;33(4):861-872. doi: 10.1016/j.arthro.2016.11.007. Epub 2017 Jan 16. https://www.ncbi.nlm.nih.gov/pubmed/28110807

Ortega-Castillo M, Medina-Porqueres I. *Effectiveness of the eccentric exercise therapy in physically active adults with symptomatic shoulder impingement or lateral epicondylar tendinopathy: A systematic review.* J Sci Med Sport. 2016 Jun;19(6):438-53. doi: 10.1016/j.jsams.2015.06.007. Epub 2015 Jun 15. https://www.ncbi.nlm.nih.gov/pubmed/26304796

Hoogvliet P, Randsdorp MS, Dingemanse R, et al. *Does effectiveness of exercise therapy and mobilisation techniques offer guidance for the treatment of lateral and medial epicondylitis?* A systematic review. Br J Sports Med. 2013 Nov;47(17):1112-9. doi: 10.1136/bjsports-2012-091990. Epub 2013 May 24. https://www.ncbi.nlm.nih.gov/pubmed/23709519

Bisset L, Coombes B, Vicenzino B. *Tennis elbow.* BMJ Clin Evid. 2011 Jun 27;2011. pii: 1117. https://www.ncbi.nlm.nih.gov/pmc/articles/pmid/21708051/

Corticosteroid References

Tan SC, Chan O. *Achilles and patellar tendinopathy: current understanding of pathophysiology and management*. Disabil Rehabil. 2008;30(20-22):1608-15. doi: 10.1080/09638280701792268. https://www.ncbi.nlm.nih.gov/pubmed/19005917

Metcalfe D, Achten J, Costa ML. *Glucocorticoid injections in lesions of the achilles tendon*. Foot Ankle Int. 2009 Jul;30(7):661-5. doi: 10.3113/FAI.2009.0661. https://www.ncbi.nlm.nih.gov/pubmed/19589313

Wiegerinck JI, Kerkhoffs GM, van Sterkenburg MN, Sierevelt IN, van Dijk CN. *Treatment for insertional Achilles tendinopathy: a systematic review*. Knee Surg Sports Traumatol Arthrosc. 2013 Jun;21(6):1345-55. doi: 10.1007/s00167-012-2219-8. Epub 2012 Oct 6. https://www.ncbi.nlm.nih.gov/pubmed/23052113

Lopez RG, Jung HG. *Achilles tendinosis: treatment options*. Clin Orthop Surg. 2015 Mar;7(1):1-7. doi: 10.4055/cios.2015.7.1.1. Epub 2015 Feb 10. https://www.ncbi.nlm.nih.gov/pmc/articles/PMC4329521/

Magnussen RA, Dunn WR, Thomson AB. *Nonoperative treatment of midportion Achilles tendinopathy: a systematic review*. Clin J Sport Med. 2009 Jan;19(1):54-64. doi: 10.1097/JSM.0b013e31818ef090. https://www.ncbi.nlm.nih.gov/pubmed/19124985

Andres BM, Murrell GA. *Treatment of tendinopathy: what works, what does not, and what is on the horizon*. Clin Orthop Relat Res. 2008 Jul;466(7):1539-54. doi: 10.1007/s11999-008-0260-1. Epub 2008 Apr 30. https://www.ncbi.nlm.nih.gov/pmc/articles/PMC2505250/

Coombes BK, Bisset L, Vicenzino B. *Efficacy and safety of corticosteroid injections and other injections for management of tendinopathy: a systematic review of randomised controlled trials*. Lancet. 2010 Nov 20;376(9754):1751-67. doi: 10.1016/S0140-6736(10)61160-9. Epub 2010 Oct 21. https://doi.org/10.1016/S0140-6736(10)61160-9

Larsson ME, Kall I, Nilsson-Helander K. *Treatment of patellar tendinopathy--a systematic review of randomized controlled trials*. Knee Surg Sports Traumatol Arthrosc. 2012 Aug;20(8):1632-46. doi: 10.1007/s00167-011-1825-1. Epub 2011 Dec 21. https://www.ncbi.nlm.nih.gov/pubmed/22186923

Saithna A, Gogna R, Baraza N, Modi C, Spencer S. *Eccentric Exercise Protocols for Patella Tendinopathy: Should we Really be Withdrawing Athletes from Sport?* Open Orthop J. 2012;6:553-7. doi: 10.2174/1874325001206010553. Epub 2012 Nov 30. https://www.ncbi.nlm.nih.gov/pmc/articles/PMC3522085/

Frizziero A, Trainito S, Oliva F, Nicoli Aldini N, Masiero S, Maffulli N. *The role of eccentric exercise in sport injuries rehabilitation*. Br Med Bull. 2014 Jun;110(1):47-75. doi: 10.1093/bmb/ldu006. Epub 2014 Apr 15. https://www.ncbi.nlm.nih.gov/pubmed/24736013

Gaujoux-Viala C, Dougados M, Gossec L. *Efficacy and safety of steroid injections for shoulder and elbow tendonitis: a meta-analysis of randomised controlled trials*. Ann Rheum Dis. 2009 Dec;68(12):1843-9. doi: 10.1136/ard.2008.099572. Epub 2008 Dec 3. https://www.ncbi.nlm.nih.gov/pmc/articles/PMC2770107/

Sims SE, Miller K, Elfar JC, Hammert WC. *Non-surgical treatment of lateral epicondylitis: a systematic review of randomized controlled trials*. Hand (N Y). 2014 Dec;9(4):419-46. doi: 10.1007/s11552-014-9642-x. https://www.ncbi.nlm.nih.gov/pmc/articles/PMC4235906/

Olaussen M, Holmedal O, Lindbaek M, et al. *Treating lateral epicondylitis with corticosteroid injections or non-electrotherapeutical physiotherapy: a systematic review*. BMJ Open 2013;3:e003564. doi: 10.1136/bmjopen-2013-003564. https://bmjopen.bmj.com/content/3/10/e003564

Arroll B, Goodyear-Smith F. *Corticosteroid injections for painful shoulder: a meta-analysis*. Br J Gen Pract. 2005 Mar;55(512):224-8. https://www.ncbi.nlm.nih.gov/pmc/articles/PMC1463095/

Greis AC, Derrington SM, McAuliffe M. *Evaluation and nonsurgical management of rotator cuff calcific tendinopathy*. Orthop Clin North Am. 2015 Apr;46(2):293-302. doi: 10.1016/j.ocl.2014.11.011. Epub 2015 Jan 27. https://jdc.jefferson.edu/cgi/viewcontent.cgi?article=1063&context=rothman_institute

Mohamadi A, Chan JJ, Claessen FM, Ring D, Chen NC. *Corticosteroid Injections Give Small and Transient Pain Relief in Rotator Cuff Tendinosis: A Meta-analysis*. Clin Orthop Relat Res. 2017 Jan;475(1):232-243. doi: 10.1007/s11999-016-5002-1. Epub 2016 Jul 28. https://www.ncbi.nlm.nih.gov/pmc/articles/PMC5174041/

Kearney RS, Parsons N, Metcalfe D, Costa ML. *Injection therapies for Achilles tendinopathy*. Cochrane Database Syst Rev. 2015 May 26;(5):CD010960. doi: 10.1002/14651858.CD010960.pub2. https://www.cochranelibrary.com/cdsr/doi/10.1002/14651858.CD010960.pub2/full

Arirachakaran A, Boonard M, Yamaphai S, et al. *Extracorporeal shock wave therapy, ultrasound-guided percutaneous lavage, corticosteroid injection and combined treatment for the treatment of rotator cuff calcific tendinopathy: a network meta-analysis of RCTs*. Eur J Orthop Surg Traumatol. 2017 Apr;27(3):381-390. doi: 10.1007/s00590-016-1839-y. Epub 2016 Aug 23. https://www.ncbi.nlm.nih.gov/pubmed/27554465

Lin MT, Chiang CF, Wu CH, et al. *Comparative Effectiveness of Injection Therapies in Rotator Cuff Tendinopathy: A Systematic Review, Pairwise and Network Meta-analysis of Randomized Controlled Trials*. Arch Phys Med Rehabil. 2019 Feb;100(2):336-349.e15. doi: 10.1016/j.apmr.2018.06.028. Epub 2018 Aug 2. https://www.ncbi.nlm.nih.gov/pubmed/30076801

Tsikopoulos K, Tsikopoulos A, Natsis K. *Autologous whole blood or corticosteroid injections for the treatment of epicondylopathy and plantar fasciopathy? A systematic review and meta-analysis of randomized controlled trials*. Phys Ther Sport. 2016 Nov;22:114-122. doi: 10.1016/j.ptsp.2016.02.002. Epub 2016 Feb 24. https://www.ncbi.nlm.nih.gov/pubmed/27085490

Dong W, Goost H, Lin XB, et al. *Injection therapies for lateral epicondylalgia: a systematic review and Bayesian network meta-analysis.* Br J Sports Med. 2016 Aug;50(15):900-8. doi: 10.1136/bjsports-2014-094387. Epub 2015 Sep 21. https://www.ncbi.nlm.nih.gov/pubmed/26392595

Maffulli N, Papalia R, D'Adamio S, et al. *Pharmacological interventions for the treatment of Achilles tendinopathy: a systematic review of randomized controlled trials.* Br Med Bull. 2015 Mar;113(1):101-15. doi: 10.1093/bmb/ldu040. Epub 2015 Jan 12. https://www.ncbi.nlm.nih.gov /pubmed/25583629

Johannsen F, Jensen S, Wetke E. *10-year follow-up after standardised treatment for Achilles tendinopathy.* BMJ Open Sport Exerc Med. 2018 Oct 4;4(1):e000415. doi: 10.1136/bmjsem-2018-000415. eCollection 2018. https://www.ncbi.nlm.nih.gov/pmc/articles/pmid/30305926/

Bisset L, Coombes B, Vicenzino B. *Tennis elbow.* BMJ Clin Evid. 2011 Jun 27;2011. pii: 1117. https://www.ncbi.nlm.nih.gov/pmc/articles /pmid/21708051/

Extracorporeal Shockwave Therapy (ECST or ECSW) References

Al-Abbad H, Simon JV. *The effectiveness of extracorporeal shock wave therapy on chronic achilles tendinopathy: a systematic review.* Foot Ankle Int. 2013 Jan;34(1):33-41. doi: 10.1177/1071100712464354. https://www.ncbi.nlm.nih.gov/pubmed/23386759

Kearney R, Costa ML. *Insertional achilles tendinopathy management: a systematic review.* Foot Ankle Int. 2010 Aug;31(8):689-94. doi: 10.3113 /FAI.2010.0689. https://www.ncbi.nlm.nih.gov/pubmed/20727317

Wiegerinck JI, Kerkhoffs GM, van Sterkenburg MN, Sierevelt IN, van Dijk CN. *Treatment for insertional Achilles tendinopathy: a systematic review.* Knee Surg Sports Traumatol Arthrosc. 2013 Jun;21(6):1345-55. doi: 10.1007/s00167-012-2219-8. Epub 2012 Oct 6. https://www. ncbi.nlm.nih.gov/pubmed/23052113

Lopez RG, Jung HG. *Achilles tendinosis: treatment options.* Clin Orthop Surg. 2015 Mar;7(1):1-7. doi: 10.4055/cios.2015.7.1.1. Epub 2015 Feb 10. https://www.ncbi.nlm.nih.gov/pmc/articles/PMC4329521/

Magnussen RA, Dunn WR, Thomson AB. *Nonoperative treatment of midportion Achilles tendinopathy: a systematic review.* Clin J Sport Med. 2009 Jan;19(1):54-64. doi: 10.1097/JSM.0b013e31818ef090. https://www.ncbi.nlm.nih.gov/pubmed/19124985

Sussmilch-Leitch SP, Collins NJ, Bialocerkowski AE, Warden SJ, Crossley KM. *Physical therapies for Achilles tendinopathy: systematic review and meta-analysis.* J Foot Ankle Res. 2012 Jul 2;5(1):15. doi: 10.1186/1757-1146-5-15. https://www.ncbi.nlm.nih.gov/pmc/articles/PMC 3537637/

Frizziero A, Trainito S, Oliva F, Nicoli Aldini N, Masiero S, Maffulli N. *The role of eccentric exercise in sport injuries rehabilitation.* Br Med Bull. 2014 Jun;110(1):47-75. doi: 10.1093/bmb/ldu006. Epub 2014 Apr 15. https://www.ncbi.nlm.nih.gov/pubmed/24736013

Mani-Babu S, Morrissey D, Waugh C, Screen H, Barton C. *The effectiveness of extracorporeal shock wave therapy in lower limb tendinopathy: a systematic review.* Am J Sports Med. 2015 Mar;43(3):752-61. doi: 10.1177/0363546514531911. Epub 2014 May 9. https://www.ncbi.nlm .nih.gov/pubmed/24817008

Korakakis V, Whiteley R, Tzavara A, Malliaropoulos N. *The effectiveness of extracorporeal shockwave therapy in common lower limb conditions: a systematic review including quantification of patient-rated pain reduction.* Br J Sports Med. 2018 Mar;52(6):387-407. doi: 10.1136/ bjsports-2016-097347. Epub 2017 Sep 27. https://bjsm.bmj.com/content/52/6/387.long

Larsson ME, Käll I, Nilsson-Helander K. *Treatment of patellar tendinopathy--a systematic review of randomized controlled trials.* Knee Surg Sports Traumatol Arthrosc. 2012 Aug;20(8):1632-46. doi: 10.1007/s00167-011-1825-1. Epub 2011 Dec 21. https://www.ncbi.nlm.nih.gov/pubmed /22186923

van der Worp H, van den Akker-Scheek I, van Schie H, Zwerver J. *ESWT for tendinopathy: technology and clinical implications.* Knee Surg Sports Traumatol Arthrosc. 2013 Jun;21(6):1451-8. doi: 10.1007/s00167-012-2009-3. Epub 2012 May 1. https://www.ncbi.nlm.nih.gov/pmc /articles/PMC3657080/

Rompe JD, Maffulli N. *Repetitive shock wave therapy for lateral elbow tendinopathy (tennis elbow): a systematic and qualitative analysis.* Br Med Bull. 2007;83:355-78. Epub 2007 Jul 11. https://www.ncbi.nlm.nih.gov/pubmed/17626054

Sims SE, Miller K, Elfar JC, Hammert WC. *Non-surgical treatment of lateral epicondylitis: a systematic review of randomized controlled trials.* Hand (N Y). 2014 Dec;9(4):419-46. doi: 10.1007/s11552-014-9642-x. https://www.ncbi.nlm.nih.gov/pmc/articles/PMC4235906/

Andres BM, Murrell GA. *Treatment of tendinopathy: what works, what does not, and what is on the horizon.* Clin Orthop Relat Res. 2008 Jul;466(7):1539-54. doi: 10.1007/s11999-008-0260-1. Epub 2008 Apr 30. https://www.ncbi.nlm.nih.gov/pmc/articles/PMC2505250/

Lee SY, Cheng B, Grimmer-Somers K. *The midterm effectiveness of extracorporeal shockwave therapy in the management of chronic calcific shoulder tendonitis.* J Shoulder Elbow Surg. 2011 Jul;20(5):845-54. doi: 10.1016/j.jse.2010.10.024. Epub 2011 Jan 13. https://www.ncbi.nlm.nih. gov/pubmed/21232988

Louwerens JK, Sierevelt IN, van Noort A, van den Bekerom MP. *Evidence for minimally invasive therapies in the management of chronic calcific tendinopathy of the rotator cuff: a systematic review and meta-analysis.* https://www.ncbi.nlm.nih.gov/pubmed/24774621

Harniman E, Carette S, Kennedy C, Beaton D. *Extracorporeal shock wave therapy for calcific and noncalcific tendonitis of the rotator cuff: a systematic review.* J Hand Ther. 2004 Apr-Jun;17(2):132-51. https://www.ncbi.nlm.nih.gov/pubmed/15162101

Greis AC, Derrington SM, McAuliffe M. *Evaluation and nonsurgical management of rotator cuff calcific tendinopathy.* Orthop Clin North Am. 2015 Apr;46(2):293-302. doi: 10.1016/j.ocl.2014.11.011. Epub 2015 Jan 27. https://jdc.jefferson.edu/cgi/viewcontent.cgi?article=1063&context=rothman_institute

Bannuru RR, Flavin NE, Vaysbrot E, Harvey W, McAlindon T. *High-energy extracorporeal shock-wave therapy for treating chronic calcific tendonitis of the shoulder: a systematic review.* Ann Intern Med. 2014 Apr 15;160(8):542-9. doi: 10.7326/M13-1982. https://www.ncbi.nlm.nih.gov/pubmed/24733195

Yu H, Randhawa K, Cote P, Optima Collaboration. *The Effectiveness of Physical Agents for Lower-Limb Soft Tissue Injuries: A Systematic Review.* J Orthop Sports Phys Ther. 2016 Jul;46(7):523-54. doi: 10.2519/jospt.2016.6521. Epub 2016 Jun 6. https://www.ncbi.nlm.nih.gov/pubmed/27266884

Louwerens JK, Veltman ES, van Noort A, van den Bekerom MP. *The Effectiveness of High-Energy Extracorporeal Shockwave Therapy Versus Ultrasound-Guided Needling Versus Arthroscopic Surgery in the Management of Chronic Calcific Rotator Cuff Tendinopathy: A Systematic Review.* Arthroscopy. 2016 Jan;32(1):165-75. doi: 10.1016/j.arthro.2015.06.049. Epub 2015 Sep 15. https://www.ncbi.nlm.nih.gov/pubmed/26382637

Wu YC, Tsai WC, Tu YK, Yu TY. *Comparative Effectiveness of Nonoperative Treatments for Chronic Calcific Tendonitis of the Shoulder: A Systematic Review and Network Meta-Analysis of Randomized Controlled Trials.* Arch Phys Med Rehabil. 2017 Aug;98(8):1678-1692.e6. doi: 10.1016/j.apmr.2017.02.030. Epub 2017 Apr 8. https://www.ncbi.nlm.nih.gov/pubmed/28400182

Startzman AN, Fowler O, Carreira D. *Proximal Hamstring Tendinosis and Partial Ruptures.* Orthopedics. 2017 Jul 1;40(4):e574-e582. doi: 10.3928/01477447-20170208-05. Epub 2017 Feb 14. https://www.ncbi.nlm.nih.gov/pubmed/28195608

Schmitz C, Csaszar NB, Milz S, et al. *Efficacy and safety of extracorporeal shock wave therapy for orthopedic conditions: a systematic review on studies listed in the PEDro database.* Br Med Bull. 2015;116:115-38. doi: 10.1093/bmb/ldv047. Epub 2015 Nov 18. https://www.ncbi.nlm.nih.gov/pmc/articles/pmid/26585999/

Bisset L, Coombes B, Vicenzino B. *Tennis elbow.* BMJ Clin Evid. 2011 Jun 27;2011. pii: 1117. https://www.ncbi.nlm.nih.gov/pmc/articles/pmid/21708051/

Low Lever Laser Therapy (LLLT) References

Nogueira AC Jr, Junior Mde J1. *The effects of laser treatment in tendinopathy: a systematic review.* Acta Ortop Bras. 2015 Jan-Feb;23(1):47-9. doi: 10.1590/1413-78522015230100513. https://www.ncbi.nlm.nih.gov/pmc/articles/pmid/26327796/

Haslerud S, Magnussen LH, Joensen J, et al. *The efficacy of low-level laser therapy for shoulder tendinopathy: a systematic review and meta-analysis of randomized controlled trials.* Physiother Res Int. 2015 Jun;20(2):108-25. doi: 10.1002/pri.1606. Epub 2014 Dec 2. https://www.ncbi.nlm.nih.gov/pubmed/25450903

Bisset L, Coombes B, Vicenzino B. *Tennis elbow.* BMJ Clin Evid. 2011 Jun 27;2011. pii: 1117. https://www.ncbi.nlm.nih.gov/pmc/articles/pmid/21708051/

Tumilty S, Munn J, McDonough S, et al. *Low level laser treatment of tendinopathy: a systematic review with meta-analysis.* Photomed Laser Surg. 2010 Feb;28(1):3-16. doi: 10.1089/pho.2008.2470. https://www.ncbi.nlm.nih.gov/pubmed/19708800

Trudel D, Duley J, Zastrow I, et al. *Rehabilitation for patients with lateral epicondylitis: a systematic review.* J Hand Ther. 2004 Apr-Jun;17(2):243-66. https://www.ncbi.nlm.nih.gov/pubmed/15162109

Sussmilch-Leitch SP, Collins NJ, Bialocerkowski AE, Warden SJ, Crossley KM. *Physical therapies for Achilles tendinopathy: systematic review and meta-analysis.* J Foot Ankle Res. 2012 Jul 2;5(1):15. doi: 10.1186/1757-1146-5-15. https://www.ncbi.nlm.nih.gov/pmc/articles/PMC3537637/

Wiegerinck JI, Kerkhoffs GM, van Sterkenburg MN, Sierevelt IN, van Dijk CN. *Treatment for insertional Achilles tendinopathy: a systematic review.* Knee Surg Sports Traumatol Arthrosc. 2013 Jun;21(6):1345-55. doi: 10.1007/s00167-012-2219-8. Epub 2012 Oct 6. https://www.ncbi.nlm.nih.gov/pubmed/23052113

Andres BM, Murrell GA. *Treatment of tendinopathy: what works, what does not, and what is on the horizon.* Clin Orthop Relat Res. 2008 Jul;466(7):1539-54. doi: 10.1007/s11999-008-0260-1. Epub 2008 Apr 30. https://www.ncbi.nlm.nih.gov/pmc/articles/pmid/18446422/

Bjordal JM, Lopes-Martins RA, Joensen J, et al. *A systematic review with procedural assessments and meta-analysis of low level laser therapy in lateral elbow tendinopathy (tennis elbow).* BMC Musculoskelet Disord. 2008 May 29;9:75. doi: 10.1186/1471-2474-9-75. https://www.ncbi.nlm.nih.gov/pmc/articles/pmid/18510742/

Desmeules F, Boudreault J, Roy JS, et al. *The efficacy of therapeutic ultrasound for rotator cuff tendinopathy: A systematic review and meta-analysis.* Phys Ther Sport. 2015 Aug;16(3):276-84. doi: 10.1016/j.ptsp.2014.09.004. Epub 2014 Sep 23. https://www.ncbi.nlm.nih.gov/pubmed/25824429

Frizziero A, Trainito S, Oliva F, et al. *The role of eccentric exercise in sport injuries rehabilitation.* Br Med Bull. 2014 Jun;110(1):47-75. doi: 10.1093/bmb/ldu006. Epub 2014 Apr 15. https://www.ncbi.nlm.nih.gov/pubmed/24736013

Platelet-Rich Plasma (PRP), Autologous blood injection (ABI), and Prolotherapy

Wang Y, Han C, Hao J, et al. *Efficacy of platelet-rich plasma injections for treating Achilles tendonitis : Systematic review of high-quality randomized controlled trials.* Orthopade. 2019 Apr 1. doi: 10.1007/s00132-019-03711-y. [Epub ahead of print]. https://www.ncbi.nlm.nih.gov/pubmed/30937491

Zhang YJ, Xu SZ, Gu PC, et al. *Is Platelet-rich Plasma Injection Effective for Chronic Achilles Tendinopathy? A Meta-analysis.* Clin Orthop Relat Res. 2018 Aug;476(8):1633-1641. doi: 10.1007/s11999.0000000000000258. https://www.ncbi.nlm.nih.gov/pubmed/29601383

Fitzpatrick J, Bulsara M, Zheng MH. *The Effectiveness of Platelet-Rich Plasma in the Treatment of Tendinopathy: A Meta-analysis of Randomized Controlled Clinical Trials.* Am J Sports Med. 2017 Jan;45(1):226-233. doi: 10.1177/0363546516643716. Epub 2016 Jul 21. https://www.ncbi.nlm.nih.gov/pubmed/27268111

Liu CJ, Yu KL, Bai JB, et al. *Platelet-rich plasma injection for the treatment of chronic Achilles tendinopathy: A meta-analysis.* Medicine (Baltimore). 2019 Apr;98(16):e15278. doi: 10.1097/MD.0000000000015278. https://www.ncbi.nlm.nih.gov/pmc/articles/pmid/31008973/

Franchini M, Cruciani M, Mengoli C, et al. *Efficacy of platelet-rich plasma as conservative treatment in orthopaedics: a systematic review and meta-analysis.* Blood Transfus. 2018 Nov;16(6):502-513. doi: 10.2450/2018.0111-18. Epub 2018 Sep 3. https://www.ncbi.nlm.nih.gov/pmc/articles/pmid/30201082/

Sandrey MA. *Autologous growth factor injections in chronic tendinopathy.* J Athl Train. 2014 May-Jun;49(3):428-30. doi: 10.4085/1062-6050-49.3.06. Epub 2014 May 19. https://www.ncbi.nlm.nih.gov/pmc/articles/pmid/24840581/

Andriolo L, Altamura SA, Reale D, et al. *Nonsurgical Treatments of Patellar Tendinopathy: Multiple Injections of Platelet-Rich Plasma Are a Suitable Option: A Systematic Review and Meta-analysis.* Am J Sports Med. 2019 Mar;47(4):1001-1018. doi: 10.1177/0363546518759674. Epub 2018 Mar 30. https://www.ncbi.nlm.nih.gov/pubmed/29601207

Chen X, Jones IA, Park C, Vangsness CT Jr. *The Efficacy of Platelet-Rich Plasma on Tendon and Ligament Healing: A Systematic Review and Meta-analysis With Bias Assessment.* Am J Sports Med. 2018 Jul;46(8):2020-2032. doi: 10.1177/0363546517743746. Epub 2017 Dec 21. https://www.ncbi.nlm.nih.gov/pubmed/29268037

Miller LE, Parrish WR, Roides B, Bhattacharyya S. *Efficacy of platelet-rich plasma injections for symptomatic tendinopathy: systematic review and meta-analysis of randomised injection-controlled trials.* BMJ Open Sport Exerc Med. 2017 Nov 6;3(1):e000237. doi: 10.1136/bmjsem-2017-000237. eCollection 2017. https://www.ncbi.nlm.nih.gov/pmc/articles/pmid/29177072/

Morath O, Kubosch EJ, Taeymans J, et al. *The effect of sclerotherapy and prolotherapy on chronic painful Achilles tendinopathy-a systematic review including meta-analysis.* Scand J Med Sci Sports. 2018 Jan;28(1):4-15. doi: 10.1111/sms.12898. Epub 2017 May 26. https://www.ncbi.nlm.nih.gov/pubmed/28449312

Filardo G, Di Matteo B, Kon E, et al. *Platelet-rich plasma in tendon-related disorders: results and indications.* Knee Surg Sports Traumatol Arthrosc. 2018 Jul;26(7):1984-1999. doi: 10.1007/s00167-016-4261-4. Epub 2016 Sep 24. https://www.ncbi.nlm.nih.gov/pubmed/27665095

Gross CE, Hsu AR, Chahal J, Holmes GB Jr. *Injectable treatments for noninsertional achilles tendinosis: a systematic review.* Foot Ankle Int. 2013 May;34(5):619-28. doi: 10.1177/1071100713475353. Epub 2013 Feb 4. https://www.ncbi.nlm.nih.gov/pubmed/23637232

Sadoghi P, Rosso C, Valderrabano V, et al. *The role of platelets in the treatment of Achilles tendon injuries.* J Orthop Res. 2013 Jan;31(1):111-8. doi: 10.1002/jor.22199. Epub 2012 Aug 6. https://www.ncbi.nlm.nih.gov/pubmed/22886696

Di Matteo B, Filardo G, Kon E, Marcacci M. *Platelet-rich plasma: evidence for the treatment of patellar and Achilles tendinopathy--a systematic review.* Musculoskelet Surg. 2015 Apr;99(1):1-9. doi: 10.1007/s12306-014-0340-1. Epub 2014 Oct 17. https://www.ncbi.nlm.nih.gov/pubmed/25323041

de Vos RJ, Windt J, Weir A. *Strong evidence against platelet-rich plasma injections for chronic lateral epicondylar tendinopathy: a systematic review.* Br J Sports Med. 2014 Jun;48(12):952-6. doi: 10.1136/bjsports-2013-093281. Epub 2014 Feb 21. https://www.ncbi.nlm.nih.gov/pubmed/24563387

Sims SE, Miller K, Elfar JC, Hammert WC. *Non-surgical treatment of lateral epicondylitis: a systematic review of randomized controlled trials.* Hand (N Y). 2014 Dec;9(4):419-46. doi: 10.1007/s11552-014-9642-x. https://www.ncbi.nlm.nih.gov/pmc/articles/pmid/25414603/

Arirachakaran A, Sukthuayat A, Sisayanarane T, et al. *Platelet-rich plasma versus autologous blood versus steroid injection in lateral epicondylitis: systematic review and network meta-analysis.* J Orthop Traumatol. 2016 Jun;17(2):101-12. doi: 10.1007/s10195-015-0376-5. Epub 2015 Sep 11. https://www.ncbi.nlm.nih.gov/pmc/articles/pmid/26362783/

Frizziero A, Trainito S, Oliva F, et al. *The role of eccentric exercise in sport injuries rehabilitation.* Br Med Bull. 2014 Jun;110(1):47-75. doi: 10.1093/bmb/ldu006. Epub 2014 Apr 15. https://www.ncbi.nlm.nih.gov/pubmed/24736013

Surgery References

Verstraelen FU, Fievez E, Janssen L, Morrenhof W. *Surgery for calcifying tendonitis of the shoulder: A systematic review.* World J Orthop. 2017 May 18;8(5):424-430. doi: 10.5312/wjo.v8.i5.424. eCollection 2017 May 18. https://www.ncbi.nlm.nih.gov/pmc/articles/pmid/28567346/

Baltes TPA, Zwiers R, Wiegerinck JI, van Dijk CN. *Surgical treatment for midportion Achilles tendinopathy: a systematic review.* Knee Surg Sports Traumatol Arthrosc. 2017 Jun;25(6):1817-1838. doi: 10.1007/s00167-016-4062-9. Epub 2016 Mar 12. https://www.ncbi.nlm.nih.gov/pmc/articles/pmid/26971111/

Brockmeyer M, Diehl N, Schmitt C, et al. *Results of Surgical Treatment of Chronic Patellar Tendinosis (Jumper's Knee): A Systematic Review of the Literature.* Arthroscopy. 2015 Dec;31(12):2424-9.e3. doi: 10.1016/j.arthro.2015.06.010. Epub 2015 Aug 3. https://www.ncbi.nlm.nih.gov/pubmed/26248496

Khan WS, Malvankar S, Bhamra JS, Pengas I. *Analysing the outcome of surgery for chronic Achilles tendinopathy over the last 50 years.* World J Orthop. 2015 Jul 18;6(6):491-7. doi: 10.5312/wjo.v6.i6.491. eCollection 2015 Jul 18. https://www.ncbi.nlm.nih.gov/pmc/articles/pmid/26191496/

Startzman AN, Fowler O, Carreira D. *Proximal Hamstring Tendinosis and Partial Ruptures.* Orthopedics. 2017 Jul 1;40(4):e574-e582. doi: 10.3928/01477447-20170208-05. Epub 2017 Feb 14. https://www.ncbi.nlm.nih.gov/pubmed/28195608

Bisset L, Coombes B, Vicenzino B. *Tennis elbow.* BMJ Clin Evid. 2011 Jun 27;2011. pii: 1117. https://www.ncbi.nlm.nih.gov/pmc/articles/pmid/21708051/

Tan SC, Chan O. *Achilles and patellar tendinopathy: current understanding of pathophysiology and management.* Disabil Rehabil. 2008;30(20-22):1608-15. doi: 10.1080/09638280701792268. https://www.ncbi.nlm.nih.gov/pubmed/19005917

Kearney R, Costa ML. *Insertional achilles tendinopathy management: a systematic review.* Foot Ankle Int. 2010 Aug;31(8):689-94. doi: 10.3113/FAI.2010.0689. https://www.ncbi.nlm.nih.gov/pubmed/20727317

Wiegerinck JI, Kerkhoffs GM, van Sterkenburg MN, Sierevelt IN, van Dijk CN. *Treatment for insertional Achilles tendinopathy: a systematic review.* Knee Surg Sports Traumatol Arthrosc. 2013 Jun;21(6):1345-55. doi: 10.1007/s00167-012-2219-8. Epub 2012 Oct 6. https://www.ncbi.nlm.nih.gov/pubmed/23052113

Larsson ME, Kall I, Nilsson-Helander K. *Treatment of patellar tendinopathy--a systematic review of randomized controlled trials.* Knee Surg Sports Traumatol Arthrosc. 2012 Aug;20(8):1632-46. doi: 10.1007/s00167-011-1825-1. Epub 2011 Dec 21. Knee Surg Sports Traumatol Arthrosc. 2012 Aug;20(8):1632-46. doi: 10.1007/s00167-011-1825-1. Epub 2011 Dec 21. https://www.ncbi.nlm.nih.gov/pubmed/22186923

Saithna A, Gogna R, Baraza N, et al. *Eccentric Exercise Protocols for Patella Tendinopathy: Should we Really be Withdrawing Athletes from Sport? A Systematic Review.* Open Orthop J. 2012;6:553-7. doi: 10.2174/1874325001206010553. Epub 2012 Nov 30. https://www.ncbi.nlm.nih.gov/pmc/articles/pmid/23248727/

Andres BM, Murrell GA. *Treatment of tendinopathy: what works, what does not, and what is on the horizon.* Clin Orthop Relat Res. 2008 Jul;466(7):1539-54. doi: 10.1007/s11999-008-0260-1. Epub 2008 Apr 30. https://www.ncbi.nlm.nih.gov/pmc/articles/pmid/18446422/

Frizziero A, Trainito S, Oliva F, et al. *The role of eccentric exercise in sport injuries rehabilitation.* Br Med Bull. 2014 Jun;110(1):47-75. doi: 10.1093/bmb/ldu006. Epub 2014 Apr 15. https://www.ncbi.nlm.nih.gov/pubmed/24736013

Ultrasound References

Dingemanse R, Randsdorp M, Koes BW, Huisstede BM. *Evidence for the effectiveness of electrophysical modalities for treatment of medial and lateral epicondylitis: a systematic review.* Br J Sports Med. 2014 Jun;48(12):957-65. doi: 10.1136/bjsports-2012-091513. Epub 2013 Jan 18. https://www.ncbi.nlm.nih.gov/pubmed/23335238

van der Windt DA1, van der Heijden GJ, van den Berg SG, et al. *Ultrasound therapy for musculoskeletal disorders: a systematic review.* Pain. 1999 Jun;81(3):257-71. https://www.ncbi.nlm.nih.gov/pubmed/10431713

Noori SA, Rasheed A, Aiyer R, et al. *Therapeutic Ultrasound for Pain Management in Chronic Low Back Pain and Chronic Neck Pain: A Systematic Review.* Pain Med. 2019 Jan 12. doi: 10.1093/pm/pny287. [Epub ahead of print]. https://www.ncbi.nlm.nih.gov/pubmed/30649460

Hoogvliet P, Randsdorp MS, Dingemanse R, et al. *Does effectiveness of exercise therapy and mobilisation techniques offer guidance for the treatment of lateral and medial epicondylitis? A systematic review.* Br J Sports Med. 2013 Nov;47(17):1112-9. doi: 10.1136/bjsports-2012-091990. Epub 2013 May 24. https://www.ncbi.nlm.nih.gov/pubmed/23709519

Bisset L, Coombes B, Vicenzino B. *Tennis elbow.* BMJ Clin Evid. 2011 Jun 27;2011. pii: 1117. https://www.ncbi.nlm.nih.gov/pmc/articles/pmid/21708051/

Trudel D, Duley J, Zastrow I, et al. *Rehabilitation for patients with lateral epicondylitis: a systematic review.* J Hand Ther. 2004 Apr-Jun;17(2):243-66. https://www.ncbi.nlm.nih.gov/pubmed/15162109

Wiegerinck JI, Kerkhoffs GM, van Sterkenburg MN, et al. *Treatment for insertional Achilles tendinopathy: a systematic review.* Knee Surg Sports Traumatol Arthrosc. 2013 Jun;21(6):1345-55. doi: 10.1007/s00167-012-2219-8. Epub 2012 Oct 6. https://www.ncbi.nlm.nih.gov/pubmed/23052113

Woodley BL, Newsham-West RJ, Baxter GD. *Chronic tendinopathy: effectiveness of eccentric exercise.* Br J Sports Med. 2007 Apr;41(4):188-98; discussion 199. Epub 2006 Oct 24. https://www.ncbi.nlm.nih.gov/pmc/articles/pmid/17062655/

Gadau M, Yeung WF, Liu H, Zaslawski C, et al. *Acupuncture and moxibustion for lateral elbow pain: a systematic review of randomized controlled trials.* BMC Complement Altern Med. 2014 Apr 12;14:136. doi: 10.1186/1472-6882-14-136. https://www.ncbi.nlm.nih.gov/pmc/articles/pmid/24726029/

Andres BM, Murrell GA. *Treatment of tendinopathy: what works, what does not, and what is on the horizon.* Clin Orthop Relat Res. 2008 Jul;466(7):1539-54. doi: 10.1007/s11999-008-0260-1. Epub 2008 Apr 30. https://www.ncbi.nlm.nih.gov/pmc/articles/pmid/18446422/

Desmeules F, Boudreault J, Roy JS, et al. *The efficacy of therapeutic ultrasound for rotator cuff tendinopathy: A systematic review and meta-analysis.* Phys Ther Sport. 2015 Aug;16(3):276-84. doi: 10.1016/j.ptsp.2014.09.004. Epub 2014 Sep 23. https://www.ncbi.nlm.nih.gov/pubmed/25824429

Greis AC, Derrington SM, McAuliffe M. *Evaluation and nonsurgical management of rotator cuff calcific tendinopathy.* Orthop Clin North Am. 2015 Apr;46(2):293-302. doi: 10.1016/j.ocl.2014.11.011. Epub 2015 Jan 27. https://www.ncbi.nlm.nih.gov/pubmed/25771323

Larsson ME, Kall I, Nilsson-Helander K. *Treatment of patellar tendinopathy--a systematic review of randomized controlled trials.* Knee Surg Sports Traumatol Arthrosc. 2012 Aug;20(8):1632-46. doi: 10.1007/s00167-011-1825-1. Epub 2011 Dec 21. Knee Surg Sports Traumatol Arthrosc. 2012 Aug;20(8):1632-46. doi: 10.1007/s00167-011-1825-1. Epub 2011 Dec 21. https://www.ncbi.nlm.nih.gov/pubmed/22186923

Wasielewski NJ, Kotsko KM. *Does eccentric exercise reduce pain and improve strength in physically active adults with symptomatic lower extremity tendinosis? A systematic review.* J Athl Train. 2007 Jul-Sep;42(3):409-21. https://www.ncbi.nlm.nih.gov/pmc/articles/pmid/18059998/

Frizziero A, Trainito S, Oliva F, et al. *The role of eccentric exercise in sport injuries rehabilitation.* Br Med Bull. 2014 Jun;110(1):47-75. doi: 10.1093/bmb/ldu006. Epub 2014 Apr 15. https://www.ncbi.nlm.nih.gov/pubmed/24736013

Botox References

Sims SE, Miller K, Elfar JC, Hammert WC. *Non-surgical treatment of lateral epicondylitis: a systematic review of randomized controlled trials.* Hand (N Y). 2014 Dec;9(4):419-46. doi: 10.1007/s11552-014-9642-x. https://www.ncbi.nlm.nih.gov/pmc/articles/pmid/25414603/

Lin YC, Wu WT, Hsu YC, et al. *Comparative effectiveness of botulinum toxin versus non-surgical treatments for treating lateral epicondylitis: a systematic review and meta-analysis.* Clin Rehabil. 2018 Feb;32(2):131-145. doi: 10.1177/0269215517702517. Epub 2017 Mar 28. https://www.ncbi.nlm.nih.gov/pubmed/28349703

Lian J, Mohamadi A, Chan JJ, et al. *Comparative Efficacy and Safety of Nonsurgical Treatment Options for Enthesopathy of the Extensor Carpi Radialis Brevis: A Systematic Review and Meta-analysis of Randomized Placebo-Controlled Trials.* Am J Sports Med. 2018 Oct 31:363546518801914. doi: 10.1177/0363546518801914. [Epub ahead of print]. https://www.ncbi.nlm.nih.gov/pubmed/30380334

Lin MT, Chiang CF, Wu CH, et al. *Comparative Effectiveness of Injection Therapies in Rotator Cuff Tendinopathy: A Systematic Review, Pairwise and Network Meta-analysis of Randomized Controlled Trials.* Arch Phys Med Rehabil. 2019 Feb;100(2):336-349.e15. doi: 10.1016/j.apmr.2018.06.028. Epub 2018 Aug 2. https://www.ncbi.nlm.nih.gov/pubmed/30076801

Kearney RS, Parsons N, Metcalfe D, Costa ML. *Injection therapies for Achilles tendinopathy.* Cochrane Database Syst Rev. 2015 May 26;(5):CD010960. doi: 10.1002/14651858.CD010960.pub2. https://www.cochranelibrary.com/cdsr/doi/10.1002/14651858.CD010960.pub2/epdf/full

Dong W, Goost H, Lin XB, et al. *Injection therapies for lateral epicondylalgia: a systematic review and Bayesian network meta-analysis.* Br J Sports Med. 2016 Aug;50(15):900-8. doi: 10.1136/bjsports-2014-094387. Epub 2015 Sep 21. https://www.ncbi.nlm.nih.gov/pubmed/26392595

Maffulli N, Papalia R, D'Adamio S2, et al. *Pharmacological interventions for the treatment of Achilles tendinopathy: a systematic review of randomized controlled trials.* Br Med Bull. 2015 Mar;113(1):101-15. doi: 10.1093/bmb/ldu040. Epub 2015 Jan 12. https://www.ncbi.nlm.nih.gov/pubmed/25583629

Ergonomics References

Dick FD, Graveling RA, Munro W, et al. *Workplace management of upper limb disorders: a systematic review.* Occup Med (Lond). 2011 Jan;61(1):19-25. doi: 10.1093/occmed/kqq174. Epub 2010 Dec 2. https://www.ncbi.nlm.nih.gov/pubmed/21127200

Stahl S, Vida D, Meisner C, et al. *Systematic review and meta-analysis on the work-related cause of de Quervain tenosynovitis: a critical appraisal of its recognition as an occupational disease.* Plast Reconstr Surg. 2013 Dec;132(6):1479-91. doi: 10.1097/01.prs.0000434409.32594.1b. https://www.ncbi.nlm.nih.gov/pubmed/24005369

van der Windt DA, Thomas E, Pope DP, et al. *Occupational risk factors for shoulder pain: a systematic review.* Occup Environ Med. 2000 Jul;57(7):433-42. https://www.ncbi.nlm.nih.gov/pmc/articles/pmid/10854494/

Iontophoresis References

Published Guidelines. Academy of Orthopaedic Physical Therapy. 15 1 2019. www.orthopt.org/content/practice/clinical-practice-guidelines addendum for mid-portion Achilles: https://www.jospt.org/doi/pdfplus/10.2519/jospt.2018.0302

Neeter C, Thomee R, Silbernagel KG, et al. *Iontophoresis with or without dexamethazone in the treatment of acute Achilles tendon pain.* Scand J Med Sci Sports. 2003 Dec;13(6):376-82. https://www.ncbi.nlm.nih.gov/pubmed/14617059

Bisset L, Coombes B, Vicenzino B. *Tennis elbow.* BMJ Clin Evid. 2011 Jun 27;2011. pii: 1117. https://www.ncbi.nlm.nih.gov/pmc/articles /pmid/21708051/

Sims SE, Miller K, Elfar JC, Hammert WC. *Non-surgical treatment of lateral epicondylitis: a systematic review of randomized controlled trials.* Hand (N Y). 2014 Dec;9(4):419-46. doi: 10.1007/s11552-014-9642-x. https://www.ncbi.nlm.nih.gov/pmc/articles/pmid/25414603/

Andres BM, Murrell GA. *Treatment of tendinopathy: what works, what does not, and what is on the horizon.* Clin Orthop Relat Res. 2008 Jul;466(7):1539-54. doi: 10.1007/s11999-008-0260-1. Epub 2008 Apr 30. https://www.ncbi.nlm.nih.gov/pmc/articles/pmid/18446422/

Magnussen RA, Dunn WR, Thomson AB. *Nonoperative treatment of midportion Achilles tendinopathy: a systematic review.* Clin J Sport Med. 2009 Jan;19(1):54-64. doi: 10.1097/JSM.0b013e31818ef090. https://www.ncbi.nlm.nih.gov/pubmed/19124985

DE Carli A, Pulcinelli F, Rose GD, et al. *Calcific tendonitis of the shoulder.* Joints. 2014 Aug 1;2(3):130-6. eCollection 2014 Jul-Sep. https://www.ncbi.nlm.nih.gov/pmc/articles/pmid/25606556/

Manual Therapy References

Desjardins-Charbonneau A, Roy JS, Dionne CE, et al. *The efficacy of manual therapy for rotator cuff tendinopathy: a systematic review and meta-analysis.* J Orthop Sports Phys Ther. 2015 May;45(5):330-50. doi: 10.2519/jospt.2015.5455. Epub 2015 Mar 26. https://www.ncbi .nlm.nih.gov/pubmed/25808530

Loew LM, Brosseau L, Tugwell P, et al. *Deep transverse friction massage for treating lateral elbow or lateral knee tendonitis.* Cochrane Database Syst Rev. 2014 Nov 8;(11):CD003528. doi: 10.1002/14651858.CD003528.pub2. https://www.ncbi.nlm.nih.gov/pubmed/25380079

Sutton D, Gross DP, Cote P, et al. *Multimodal care for the management of musculoskeletal disorders of the elbow, forearm, wrist and hand: a systematic review by the Ontario Protocol for Traffic Injury Management (OPTIMa) Collaboration.* Chiropr Man Therap. 2016 Mar 7;24:8. doi: 10.1186/s12998-016-0089-8. eCollection 2016. https://www.ncbi.nlm.nih.gov/pmc/articles/pmid/26955466/

Olaussen M, Holmedal O, Lindbaek M, et al. *Treating lateral epicondylitis with corticosteroid injections or non-electrotherapeutical physiotherapy: a systematic review.* BMJ Open. 2013 Oct 29;3(10):e003564. doi: 10.1136/bmjopen-2013-003564. https://www.ncbi.nlm.nih.gov/pmc/ articles/pmid/24171937/

Hoogvliet P, Randsdorp MS, Dingemanse R, et al. *Does effectiveness of exercise therapy and mobilisation techniques offer guidance for the treatment of lateral and medial epicondylitis? A systematic review.* Br J Sports Med. 2013 Nov;47(17):1112-9. doi: 10.1136/bjsports-2012-091990. Epub 2013 May 24. https://www.ncbi.nlm.nih.gov/pubmed/23709519

Joseph MF, Taft K, Moskwa M, Denegar CR. *Deep friction massage to treat tendinopathy: a systematic review of a classic treatment in the face of a new paradigm of understanding.* J Sport Rehabil. 2012 Nov;21(4):343-53. Epub 2011 Dec 30. https://www.ncbi.nlm.nih.gov/pubmed /22234925

Hawk C, Minkalis AL, Khorsan R, et al. *Systematic Review of Nondrug, Nonsurgical Treatment of Shoulder Conditions.* J Manipulative Physiol Ther. 2017 Jun;40(5):293-319. doi: 10.1016/j.jmpt.2017.04.001. Epub 2017 May 26. https://www.ncbi.nlm.nih.gov/pubmed/28554433

Page MJ, Green S, McBain B, et al. *Manual therapy and exercise for rotator cuff disease.* Cochrane Database Syst Rev. 2016 Jun 10;(6):CD012224. doi: 10.1002/14651858.CD012224. https://www.ncbi.nlm.nih.gov/pubmed/27283590

Brosseau L, Casimiro L, Milne S, et al. *Deep transverse friction massage for treating tendonitis.* Cochrane Database Syst Rev. 2002;(4):CD003528. https://www.ncbi.nlm.nih.gov/pubmed/12519601

Bisset L, Coombes B, Vicenzino B. *Tennis elbow.* BMJ Clin Evid. 2011 Jun 27;2011. pii: 1117. https://www.ncbi.nlm.nih.gov/pmc/articles/pmid /21708051/

Hoogvliet P, Randsdorp MS, Dingemanse R, et al. *Does effectiveness of exercise therapy and mobilisation techniques offer guidance for the treatment of lateral and medial epicondylitis? A systematic review.* Br J Sports Med. 2013 Nov;47(17):1112-9. doi: 10.1136/bjsports-2012-091990. Epub 2013 May 24. https://www.ncbi.nlm.nih.gov/pubmed/23709519

Chughtai M, Newman JM, Sultan AA, et al. *Astym® therapy: a systematic review.* Ann Transl Med. 2019 Feb;7(4):70. doi: 10.21037/atm.2018.11.49. https://www.ncbi.nlm.nih.gov/pmc/articles/pmid/30963065/

Cheatham SW, Lee M, Cain M, Baker R. *The efficacy of instrument assisted soft tissue mobilization: a systematic review.* J Can Chiropr Assoc. 2016 Sep;60(3):200-211. https://www.ncbi.nlm.nih.gov/pmc/articles/pmid/27713575/

Needling Techniques (Acupuncture, dry needling, etc.) References

Cox J, Varatharajan S, Cote P, Optima Collaboration. *Effectiveness of Acupuncture Therapies to Manage Musculoskeletal Disorders of the Extremities: A Systematic Review.* J Orthop Sports Phys Ther. 2016 Jun;46(6):409-29. doi: 10.2519/jospt.2016.6270. Epub 2016 Apr 26. https://www.jospt.org/doi/full/10.2519/jospt.2016.6270

Krey D, Borchers J, McCamey K. *Tendon needling for treatment of tendinopathy: A systematic review.* Phys Sportsmed. 2015 Feb;43(1):80-6. doi: 10.1080/00913847.2015.1004296. Epub 2015 Jan 22. https://www.ncbi.nlm.nih.gov/pubmed/25613418

Green S, Buchbinder R, Hetrick S. *Acupuncture for shoulder pain.* Cochrane Database Syst Rev. 2005 Apr 18;(2):CD005319. https://www.ncbi.nlm.nih.gov/pubmed/15846753

Trudel D, Duley J, Zastrow I, et al. *Rehabilitation for patients with lateral epicondylitis: a systematic review.* J Hand Ther. 2004 Apr-Jun;17(2):243-66. https://www.ncbi.nlm.nih.gov/pubmed/15162109

Trinh KV, Phillips SD, Ho E, Damsma K. *Acupuncture for the alleviation of lateral epicondyle pain: a systematic review.* Rheumatology (Oxford). 2004 Sep;43(9):1085-90. Epub 2004 Jun 22. https://www.ncbi.nlm.nih.gov/pubmed/15213328

Grant HJ, Arthur A, Pichora DR. *Evaluation of interventions for rotator cuff pathology: a systematic review.* J Hand Ther. 2004 Apr-Jun;17(2):274-99. https://www.ncbi.nlm.nih.gov/pubmed/15162111

Green S, Buchbinder R, Barnsley L, et al. *Acupuncture for lateral elbow pain.* Cochrane Database Syst Rev. 2002;(1):CD003527. https://www.ncbi.nlm.nih.gov/pubmed/11869671

Chang WD, Lai PT, Tsou YA. *Analgesic effect of manual acupuncture and laser acupuncture for lateral epicondylalgia: a systematic review and meta-analysis.* Am J Chin Med. 2014;42(6):1301-14. doi: 10.1142/S0192415X14500815. https://www.ncbi.nlm.nih.gov/pubmed/25384448

Mendonca LM, Leite HR, Zwerver J, et al. *How strong is the evidence that conservative treatment reduces pain and improves function in individuals with patellar tendinopathy? A systematic review of randomised controlled trials including GRADE recommendations.* Br J Sports Med. 2019 Jun 6. pii: bjsports-2018-099747. doi: 10.1136/bjsports-2018-099747. [Epub ahead of print]. https://www.ncbi.nlm.nih.gov/pubmed/31171514

Frizziero A, Trainito S, Oliva F, et al. *The role of eccentric exercise in sport injuries rehabilitation.* Br Med Bull. 2014 Jun;110(1):47-75. doi: 10.1093/bmb/ldu006. Epub 2014 Apr 15. https://www.ncbi.nlm.nih.gov/pubmed/24736013

Woitzik E, Jacobs C, Wong JJ, et al. *The effectiveness of exercise on recovery and clinical outcomes of soft tissue injuries of the leg, ankle, and foot: A systematic review by the Ontario Protocol for Traffic Injury Management (OPTIMa) Collaboration.* Man Ther. 2015 Oct;20(5):633-45. doi: 10.1016/j.math.2015.03.012. Epub 2015 Mar 28. https://www.ncbi.nlm.nih.gov/pubmed/25892707

Gadau M, Yeung WF, Liu H, et al. *Acupuncture and moxibustion for lateral elbow pain: a systematic review of randomized controlled trials.* BMC Complement Altern Med. 2014 Apr 12;14:136. doi: 10.1186/1472-6882-14-136. https://www.ncbi.nlm.nih.gov/pmc/articles/pmid/24726029/

Bisset L, Coombes B, Vicenzino B. *Tennis elbow.* BMJ Clin Evid. 2011 Jun 27;2011. pii: 1117. https://www.ncbi.nlm.nih.gov/pmc/articles/pmid/21708051/

Nitroglycerine/Nitric Oxide/Glyceryl Trinitrate (GTN) References

Challoumas D, Kirwan PD, Borysov D, et al. *Topical glyceryl trinitrate for the treatment of tendinopathies: a systematic review.* Br J Sports Med. 2019 Feb;53(4):251-262. doi: 10.1136/bjsports-2018-099552. Epub 2018 Oct 9. https://www.ncbi.nlm.nih.gov/pmc/articles/pmid/30301735/

Maffulli N, Papalia R, D'Adamio S, et al. *Pharmacological interventions for the treatment of Achilles tendinopathy: a systematic review of randomized controlled trials.* Br Med Bull. 2015 Mar;113(1):101-15. doi: 10.1093/bmb/ldu040. Epub 2015 Jan 12. https://www.ncbi.nlm.nih.gov/pubmed/25583629

Gambito ED, Gonzalez-Suarez CB, Oquinena TI, Agbayani RB. *Evidence on the effectiveness of topical nitroglycerin in the treatment of tendinopathies: a systematic review and meta-analysis.* Arch Phys Med Rehabil. 2010 Aug;91(8):1291-305. doi: 10.1016/j.apmr.2010.02.008. https://www.ncbi.nlm.nih.gov/pubmed/20684913

Cumpston M, Johnston RV, Wengier L, Buchbinder R. *Topical glyceryl trinitrate for rotator cuff disease.* Cochrane Database Syst Rev. 2009 Jul 8;(3):CD006355. doi: 10.1002/14651858.CD006355.pub2. https://www.ncbi.nlm.nih.gov/pubmed/19588386

Andres BM, Murrell GA. *Treatment of tendinopathy: what works, what does not, and what is on the horizon.* Clin Orthop Relat Res. 2008 Jul;466(7):1539-54. doi: 10.1007/s11999-008-0260-1. Epub 2008 Apr 30. https://www.ncbi.nlm.nih.gov/pmc/articles/pmid/18446422/

McCallum SD, Paoloni JA, Murrell GA. *Five-year prospective comparison study of topical glyceryl trinitrate treatment of chronic lateral epicondylosis at the elbow.* Br J Sports Med. 2011 Apr;45(5):416-20. doi: 10.1136/bjsm.2009.061002. Epub 2009 Jun 23. https://www.ncbi.nlm.nih.gov/pubmed/19553221

Pain Medication References

Pattanittum P, Turner T, Green S, Buchbinder R. *Non-steroidal anti-inflammatory drugs (NSAIDs) for treating lateral elbow pain in adults.* Cochrane Database Syst Rev. 2013 May 31;(5):CD003686. doi: 10.1002/14651858.CD003686.pub2. https://www.ncbi.nlm.nih.gov/pubmed/23728646

Tan SC, Chan O. *Achilles and patellar tendinopathy: current understanding of pathophysiology and management.* Disabil Rehabil. 2008;30(20-22):1608-15. doi: 10.1080/09638280701792268. https://www.ncbi.nlm.nih.gov/pubmed/19005917

Frizziero A, Trainito S, Oliva F, et al. *The role of eccentric exercise in sport injuries rehabilitation.* Br Med Bull. 2014 Jun;110(1):47-75. doi: 10.1093/bmb/ldu006. Epub 2014 Apr 15. https://www.ncbi.nlm.nih.gov/pubmed/24736013

Gaujoux-Viala C, Dougados M, Gossec L. *Efficacy and safety of steroid injections for shoulder and elbow tendonitis: a meta-analysis of randomised controlled trials.* Ann Rheum Dis. 2009 Dec;68(12):1843-9. doi: 10.1136/ard.2008.099572. Epub 2008 Dec 3. https://www.ncbi.nlm.nih.gov/pmc/articles/pmid/19054817/

Gadau M, Yeung WF, Liu H, et al. *Acupuncture and moxibustion for lateral elbow pain: a systematic review of randomized controlled trials.* BMC Complement Altern Med. 2014 Apr 12;14:136. doi: 10.1186/1472-6882-14-136. https://www.ncbi.nlm.nih.gov/pmc/articles/pmid/24726029/

Arroll B, Goodyear-Smith F. *Corticosteroid injections for painful shoulder: a meta-analysis.* Br J Gen Pract. 2005 Mar;55(512):224-8. https://www.ncbi.nlm.nih.gov/pmc/articles/pmid/15808040/

Bisset L, Coombes B, Vicenzino B. *Tennis elbow.* BMJ Clin Evid. 2011 Jun 27;2011. pii: 1117. https://www.ncbi.nlm.nih.gov/pmc/articles/pmid/21708051/

Trappe TA, White F, Lambert CP, Cesar D. *Effect of ibuprofen and acetaminophen on postexercise muscle protein synthesis.* Am J Physiol Endocrinol Metab. 2002 Mar;282(3):E551-6. https://www.ncbi.nlm.nih.gov/pubmed/11832356

Lundberg TR, Howatson G. *Analgesic and anti-inflammatory drugs in sports: Implications for exercise performance and training adaptations.* Scand J Med Sci Sports. 2018 Nov;28(11):2252-2262. doi: 10.1111/sms.13275. Epub 2018 Sep 2. https://www.ncbi.nlm.nih.gov/pubmed/30102811

Stretching References

Published Guidelines. Academy of Orthopaedic Physical Therapy. 15 1 2019. www.orthopt.org/content/practice/clinical-practice-guidelines addendum for mid-portion Achilles: https://www.jospt.org/doi/pdfplus/10.2519/jospt.2018.0302

Hoogvliet P, Randsdorp MS, Dingemanse R, et al. *Does effectiveness of exercise therapy and mobilisation techniques offer guidance for the treatment of lateral and medial epicondylitis? A systematic review.* Br J Sports Med. 2013 Nov;47(17):1112-9. doi: 10.1136/bjsports-2012-091990. Epub 2013 May 24. https://www.ncbi.nlm.nih.gov/pubmed/23709519

Desjardins-Charbonneau A, Roy JS, Dionne CE, Desmeules F. *THE EFFICACY OF TAPING FOR ROTATOR CUFF TENDINOPATHY: A SYSTEMATIC REVIEW AND META-ANALYSIS.* Int J Sports Phys Ther. 2015 Aug;10(4):420-33. https://www.ncbi.nlm.nih.gov/pmc/articles/pmid/26346114/

Witvrouw E, Mahieu N, Roosen P, McNair P. *The role of stretching in tendon injuries.* Br J Sports Med. 2007 Apr;41(4):224-6. Epub 2007 Jan 29. https://www.ncbi.nlm.nih.gov/pmc/articles/pmid/17261561/

McHugh MP, Cosgrave CH. *To stretch or not to stretch: the role of stretching in injury prevention and performance.* Scand J Med Sci Sports. 2010 Apr;20(2):169-81. doi: 10.1111/j.1600-0838.2009.01058.x. Epub 2009 Dec 18. https://www.ncbi.nlm.nih.gov/pubmed/20030776/

Sutton D, Gross DP, Cote P, et al. *Multimodal care for the management of musculoskeletal disorders of the elbow, forearm, wrist and hand: a systematic review by the Ontario Protocol for Traffic Injury Management (OPTIMa) Collaboration.* Chiropr Man Therap. 2016 Mar 7;24:8. doi: 10.1186/s12998-016-0089-8. eCollection 2016. https://www.ncbi.nlm.nih.gov/pmc/articles/pmid/26955466/

Desjardins-Charbonneau A, Roy JS, Dionne CE, et al. *The efficacy of manual therapy for rotator cuff tendinopathy: a systematic review and meta-analysis.* J Orthop Sports Phys Ther. 2015 May;45(5):330-50. doi: 10.2519/jospt.2015.5455. Epub 2015 Mar 26. https://www.ncbi.nlm.nih.gov/pubmed/25808530

Woodley BL, Newsham-West RJ, Baxter GD. *Chronic tendinopathy: effectiveness of eccentric exercise.* Br J Sports Med. 2007 Apr;41(4):188-98; discussion 199. Epub 2006 Oct 24. https://www.ncbi.nlm.nih.gov/pmc/articles/pmid/17062655/

Supplements References

Lewis JS, Sandford FM. *Rotator cuff tendinopathy: is there a role for polyunsaturated Fatty acids and antioxidants?* J Hand Ther. 2009 Jan-Mar;22(1):49-55; quiz 56. doi: 10.1197/j.jht.2008.06.007. Epub 2008 Aug 30. https://www.ncbi.nlm.nih.gov/pubmed/18950988

Fusini F, Bisicchia S, Bottegoni C, et al. *Nutraceutical supplement in the management of tendinopathies: a systematic review.* Muscles Ligaments Tendons J. 2016 May 19;6(1):48-57. doi: 10.11138/mltj/2016.6.1.048. eCollection 2016 Jan-Mar. https://www.ncbi.nlm.nih.gov/pmc/articles/pmid/27331031/

DePhillipo NN, Aman ZS, Kennedy MI, et al. *Efficacy of Vitamin C Supplementation on Collagen Synthesis and Oxidative Stress After Musculoskeletal Injuries: A Systematic Review.* Orthop J Sports Med. 2018 Oct 25;6(10):2325967118804544. doi: 10.1177/2325967118804544. eCollection 2018 Oct.

Tack C, Shorthouse F, Kass L. *The Physiological Mechanisms of Effect of Vitamins and Amino Acids on Tendon and Muscle Healing: A Systematic Review.* Int J Sport Nutr Exerc Metab. 2018 May 1;28(3):294-311. doi: 10.1123/ijsnem.2017-0267. Epub 2018 Jun 1. https://www.ncbi.nlm.nih.gov/pubmed/29140140

Page MJ, Green S, McBain B, et al. *Manual therapy and exercise for rotator cuff disease.* Cochrane Database Syst Rev. 2016 Jun 10;(6):CD012224. doi: 10.1002/14651858.CD012224. https://www.ncbi.nlm.nih.gov/pubmed/27283590

Shaw G, Lee-Barthel A, Ross ML, et al. *Vitamin C-enriched gelatin supplementation before intermittent activity augments collagen synthesis.* Am J Clin Nutr. 2017 Jan;105(1):136-143. doi: 10.3945/ajcn.116.138594. Epub 2016 Nov 16. https://www.ncbi.nlm.nih.gov/pmc/articles/pmid/27852613/

Praet SFE, Purdam CR, Welvaert M, et al. *Oral Supplementation of Specific Collagen Peptides Combined with Calf-Strengthening Exercises Enhances Function and Reduces Pain in Achilles Tendinopathy Patients.* Nutrients. 2019 Jan 2;11(1). pii: E76. doi: 10.3390/nu11010076. https://www.ncbi.nlm.nih.gov/pmc/articles/pmid/30609761/

Lis DM, Baar K. Effects of Different Vitamin C-Enriched Collagen Derivatives on Collagen Synthesis. Int J Sport Nutr Exerc Metab. 2019 Jun 6:1-6. doi: 10.1123/ijsnem.2018-0385. [Epub ahead of print]. https://www.ncbi.nlm.nih.gov/pubmed/30859848

Abate M, Schiavone C, Salini V. *The use of hyaluronic acid after tendon surgery and in tendinopathies.* Biomed Res Int. 2014;2014:783632. doi: 10.1155/2014/783632. Epub 2014 May 8. https://www.ncbi.nlm.nih.gov/pmc/articles/pmid/24895610/

Kaux JF, Samson A, Crielaard JM. *Hyaluronic acid and tendon lesions.* Muscles Ligaments Tendons J. 2016 Feb 13;5(4):264-9. doi: 10.11138/mltj/2015.5.4.264. eCollection 2015 Oct-Dec. https://www.ncbi.nlm.nih.gov/pmc/articles/pmid/26958533/

Russell JE, Manske PR. *Ascorbic acid requirement for optimal flexor tendon repair in vitro.* J Orthop Res. 1991 Sep;9(5):714-9. https://www.ncbi.nlm.nih.gov/pubmed/1870035

Omeroglu S, Peker T, Turkozkan N, Omeroglu H. *High-dose vitamin C supplementation accelerates the Achilles tendon healing in healthy rats.* Arch Orthop Trauma Surg. 2009 Feb;129(2):281-6. doi: 10.1007/s00402-008-0603-0. Epub 2008 Feb 29. https://www.ncbi.nlm.nih.gov/pubmed/18309503

Melendez-Hevia E, De Paz-Lugo P, Cornish-Bowden A, Cardenas ML. *A weak link in metabolism: the metabolic capacity for glycine biosynthesis does not satisfy the need for collagen synthesis.* J Biosci. 2009 Dec;34(6):853-72.

Kalman DS. *Amino Acid Composition of an Organic Brown Rice Protein Concentrate and Isolate Compared to Soy and Whey Concentrates and Isolates.* Foods. 2014 Jun 30;3(3):394-402. doi: 10.3390/foods3030394. https://www.ncbi.nlm.nih.gov/pmc/articles/pmid/28234326/

Eastoe JE. *The amino acid composition of mammalian collagen and gelatin.* Biochem J. 1955 Dec;61(4):589-600. https://www.ncbi.nlm.nih.gov/pmc/articles/pmid/13276342/

Sigma Nutrition. *SNR #143: Keith Baar, PhD – Tendon Stiffness, Collagen Production & Gelatin for Performance & Injury podcast.* 2019. [online] Available at: http://sigmanutrition.com/episode143/ [Accessed 25 June 2019].

Oryan A, Moshiri A, Meimandiparizi AH. Effects of sodium-hyaluronate and glucosamine-chondroitin sulfate on remodeling stage of tenotomized superficial digital flexor tendon in rabbits: a clinical, histopathological, ultrastructural, and biomechanical study. Connect Tissue Res. 2011;52(4):329-39. doi: 10.3109/03008207.2010.531332. Epub 2010 Nov 30. https://www.ncbi.nlm.nih.gov/pubmed/21117902

Flores C, Balius R, Álvarez G, et al. Efficacy and Tolerability of Peritendinous Hyaluronic Acid in Patients with Supraspinatus Tendinopathy: a Multicenter, Randomized, Controlled Trial. Sports Med Open. 2017 Dec;3(1):22. doi: 10.1186/s40798-017-0089-9. Epub 2017 Jun 5. https://www.ncbi.nlm.nih.gov/pmc/articles/pmid/28585109/

TENS (Transcutaneous Electrical Nerve Stimulation) References

Desmeules F1, Boudreault J2, Roy JS, et al. *Efficacy of transcutaneous electrical nerve stimulation for rotator cuff tendinopathy: a systematic review.* Physiotherapy. 2016 Mar;102(1):41-9. doi: 10.1016/j.physio.2015.06.004. Epub 2015 Sep 7. https://www.ncbi.nlm.nih.gov/pubmed/26619821

Page MJ, Green S, Mrocki MA, et al. *Electrotherapy modalities for rotator cuff disease.* Cochrane Database Syst Rev. 2016 Jun 10;(6):CD012225. doi: 10.1002/14651858.CD012225. https://www.ncbi.nlm.nih.gov/pubmed/27283591

Dingemanse R, Randsdorp M, Koes BW, Huisstede BM. *Evidence for the effectiveness of electrophysical modalities for treatment of medial and lateral epicondylitis: a systematic review.* Br J Sports Med. 2014 Jun;48(12):957-65. doi: 10.1136/bjsports-2012-091513. Epub 2013 Jan 18. https://www.ncbi.nlm.nih.gov/pubmed/23335238

Machado AF, Santana EF, Tacani PM, Liebano RE. *The effects of transcutaneous electrical nerve stimulation on tissue repair: A literature review.* Can J Plast Surg. 2012 Winter;20(4):237-40. https://www.ncbi.nlm.nih.gov/pmc/articles/pmid/24294017/

Wait and see (or watchful waiting) References

Sims SE, Miller K, Elfar JC, Hammert WC. *Non-surgical treatment of lateral epicondylitis: a systematic review of randomized controlled trials.* Hand (N Y). 2014 Dec;9(4):419-46. doi: 10.1007/s11552-014-9642-x. https://www.ncbi.nlm.nih.gov/pmc/articles/pmid/25414603/

Menta R, Randhawa K, Cote P, et al. *The effectiveness of exercise for the management of musculoskeletal disorders and injuries of the elbow, forearm, wrist, and hand: a systematic review by the Ontario Protocol for Traffic Injury Management (OPTIMa) collaboration.* J Manipulative Physiol Ther. 2015 Sep;38(7):507-20. doi: 10.1016/j.jmpt.2015.06.002. Epub 2015 Jun 27. https://www.ncbi.nlm.nih.gov/pubmed/26130104

Sayegh ET, Strauch RJ. *Does nonsurgical treatment improve longitudinal outcomes of lateral epicondylitis over no treatment? A meta-analysis.* Clin Orthop Relat Res. 2015 Mar;473(3):1093-107. doi: 10.1007/s11999-014-4022-y. Epub 2014 Oct 29. https://www.ncbi.nlm.nih.gov/pmc/articles/pmid/25352261/

Barr S, Cerisola FL, Blanchard V. *Effectiveness of corticosteroid injections compared with physiotherapeutic interventions for lateral epicondylitis: a systematic review.* Physiotherapy. 2009 Dec;95(4):251-65. doi: 10.1016/j.physio.2009.05.002. Epub 2009 Jul 24. https://www.ncbi.nlm.nih.gov/pubmed/19892089

Frizziero A, Trainito S, Oliva F. *The role of eccentric exercise in sport injuries rehabilitation.* Br Med Bull. 2014 Jun;110(1):47-75. doi: 10.1093/bmb/ldu006. Epub 2014 Apr 15. https://www.ncbi.nlm.nih.gov/pubmed/24736013

Gaujoux-Viala C, Dougados M, Gossec L. *Efficacy and safety of steroid injections for shoulder and elbow tendonitis: a meta-analysis of randomised controlled trials.* Ann Rheum Dis. 2009 Dec;68(12):1843-9. doi: 10.1136/ard.2008.099572. Epub 2008 Dec 3. https://www.ncbi.nlm.nih.gov/pmc/articles/pmid/19054817/

Calcific Tendinopathy References

ElShewy MT. *Calcific tendonitis of the rotator cuff.* World J Orthop. 2016 Jan 18;7(1):55-60. doi: 10.5312/wjo.v7.i1.55. eCollection 2016 Jan 18. https://www.ncbi.nlm.nih.gov/pmc/articles/pmid/26807357/

Zhang T, Duan Y, Chen J, Chen X. *Efficacy of ultrasound-guided percutaneous lavage for rotator cuff calcific tendinopathy: A systematic review and meta-analysis.* Medicine (Baltimore). 2019 May;98(21):e15552. doi: 10.1097/MD.0000000000015552. https://www.ncbi.nlm.nih.gov/pmc/articles/pmid/31124934/

Lafrance S, Doiron-Cadrin P, Saulnier M, et al. *Is ultrasound-guided lavage an effective intervention for rotator cuff calcific tendinopathy? A systematic review with a meta-analysis of randomised controlled trials.* BMJ Open Sport Exerc Med. 2019 Mar 9;5(1):e000506. doi: 10.1136/bmjsem-2018-000506. eCollection 2019. https://www.ncbi.nlm.nih.gov/pmc/articles/pmid/31191964/

Wu YC, Tsai WC, Tu YK, Yu TY. *Comparative Effectiveness of Nonoperative Treatments for Chronic Calcific Tendinitis of the Shoulder: A Systematic Review and Network Meta-Analysis of Randomized Controlled Trials.* Arch Phys Med Rehabil. 2017 Aug;98(8):1678-1692.e6. doi: 10.1016/j.apmr.2017.02.030. Epub 2017 Apr 8. https://www.ncbi.nlm.nih.gov/pubmed/28400182

Louwerens JK, Sierevelt IN, van Noort A, van den Bekerom MP. *Evidence for minimally invasive therapies in the management of chronic calcific tendinopathy of the rotator cuff: a systematic review and meta-analysis.* J Shoulder Elbow Surg. 2014 Aug;23(8):1240-9. doi: 10.1016/j.jse.2014.02.002. Epub 2014 Apr 26. https://www.ncbi.nlm.nih.gov/pubmed/24774621

Verstraelen FU, In den Kleef NJ, Jansen L, Morrenhof JW. *High-energy versus low-energy extracorporeal shock wave therapy for calcifying tendinitis of the shoulder: which is superior? A meta-analysis.* Clin Orthop Relat Res. 2014 Sep;472(9):2816-25. doi: 10.1007/s11999-014-3680-0. Epub 2014 May 29. https://www.ncbi.nlm.nih.gov/pmc/articles/pmid/24872197/

Ioppolo F, Tattoli M, Di Sante L, et al. *Clinical improvement and resorption of calcifications in calcific tendonitis of the shoulder after shock wave therapy at 6 months' follow-up: a systematic review and meta-analysis.* Arch Phys Med Rehabil. 2013 Sep;94(9):1699-706. doi: 10.1016/j.apmr.2013.01.030. Epub 2013 Mar 13. https://www.ncbi.nlm.nih.gov/pubmed/23499780

Hawk C, Minkalis AL, Khorsan R, et al. *Systematic Review of Nondrug, Nonsurgical Treatment of Shoulder Conditions.* J Manipulative Physiol Ther. 2017 Jun;40(5):293-319. doi: 10.1016/j.jmpt.2017.04.001. Epub 2017 May 26. https://www.ncbi.nlm.nih.gov/pubmed/28554433

Printed in Great Britain
by Amazon

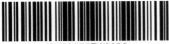